Gut feelings: An informative guide to living with Crohn's Disease and Ulcerative Colitis

Navigate Your Way Through These Autoimmune Diseases

Séamus John Power

Power- Dowie Publishing

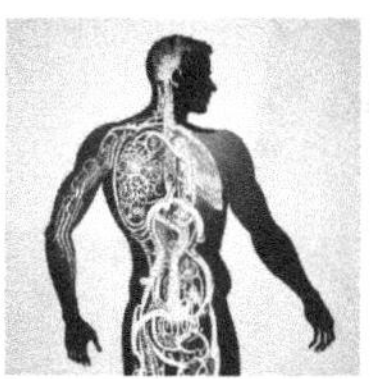

© Copyright 2024 - All rights reserved.

The content contained within this book may not be reproduced, duplicated, or transmitted without direct written permission from the author or the publisher.

Under no circumstances will any blame or legal responsibility be held against the publisher, or author, for any damages, reparation, or monetary loss due to the information contained within this book, either directly or indirectly.

<u>Legal Notice:</u>

This book is copyright protected. It is only for personal use. You cannot amend, distribute, sell, use, quote or paraphrase any part, or the content within this book, without the consent of the author or publisher.

<u>Disclaimer Notice:</u>

Contents

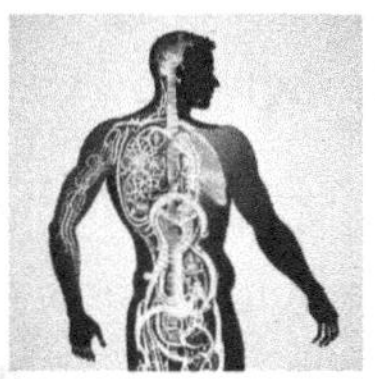

Introduction

Hello there! I'm Séamus John Power, an author and fitness instructor. In 2012, I was hit with a life-altering diagnosis: ulcerative colitis, targeting my lower colon. This book was born from my desire to support anyone newly diagnosed or journeying with Crohn's or colitis. Think of it as your trusty companion on this unpredictable path, offering encouragement, advice, and maybe a few laughs along the way.

Let me be real—my journey has had more twists and turns than a roller coaster. At first, I brushed off my symptoms—blood, mucus, intense bowel issues, and relentless cramps—as if they were no big deal. I charged on, pretending all was well until reality struck hard one day during an exercise class. I lost control of my bowels in front of my students, and that embarrassing wake-up call finally sent me to seek medical help. A colonoscopy later, I was officially diagnosed with pan colitis. Thankfully, there was no scarring; just a couple of polyps were removed on the spot.

I started on mesalazine tablets, which worked wonders for about a year. But when my symptoms returned, even with a higher dose, it was clear I was in for a battle. Suppositories brought relief for a while, and I felt like I'd found remission. But Christmas 2016 delivered a painful flare-up. Steroids helped manage it, though they weren't exactly my best friends. Then I was introduced to Entyvio (vedolizumab), a biologic given through infusions every six weeks. This helped for a solid year until I switched to a self-injecting pen, which didn't work as well. So, I went back to hospital infusions—this time, every four weeks, at the maximum dose. Thankfully, I've now been in remission for almost five years, with only occasional flare-ups that mesalazine suppositories quickly calm.

Throughout it all, exercise has been my mental rock. I teach everything from high-intensity workouts to yoga and Pilates. I've had only one close call during class, and my students still joke about how they saw me dash to the restroom at lightning speed. And yes, there was one memorable car mishap—what can you do but laugh?

Diet has been another crucial factor. I adore spicy food, but it doesn't exactly love me back! A touch of spice I can handle, but I know my limits. And alcohol—well, a drink here and there is fine, but I've learned overindulgence can spell trouble.

My hope for you as you read this book is that you feel less alone and more empowered. With this guide, I aim to share the insights and strategies that have worked for me. Living with Crohn's or colitis may not be easy, but there is always hope.

Here's to navigating this journey together,

Séamus.

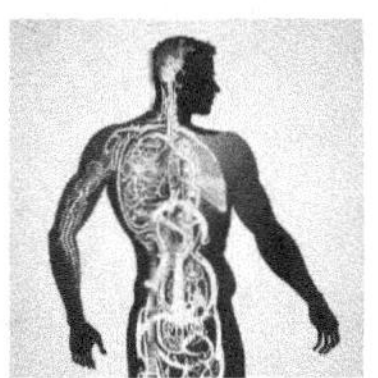

Chapter 1: Meet Your Microbiome: The Gut Squad

Your gut is more than just a place where food is broken down. It's home to an entire ecosystem that plays a key role in keeping your body balanced. Inside your gut, you have a group of microbiomes composed of bacteria, fungi, and other microorganisms. We can call these your "gut squad."

As you explore this chapter, you'll learn what the microbiome is and how it affects your immune function and digestion, two crucial systems in maintaining health. You'll discover the importance of a balanced microbiome, what factors can tip the scales, and how such imbalances influence autoimmune conditions. Whether living with an autoimmune disease, supporting a loved one, or advising clients as a health professional, this chapter offers practical advice, relatable insights, and a nod to humor, ensuring you leave with valuable tools for navigating daily life with optimism and resilience.

Gut Microbes and Digestion

The gut is home to trillions of bacteria, collectively known as the microbiome, which influence digestion and our body's immune responses. These microscopic inhabitants are active participants in managing our health.

Your gut squad can be roughly divided into two camps: the "good guys" and the "not-so-good guys." The good guys are bacteria such as *Lactobacillus* and *Bifidobacterium*; these are the health enthusiasts of your microbiome, working hard to keep things running smoothly. They help break down complex foods, release important nutrients, and protect your gut lining from unwanted invaders. The not-so-good guys, however, are always lurking. While a few of them serve useful purposes, too many can trigger chaos, creating symptoms and problems that can irritate your gut, causing digestive problems.

How the Microbiome Supports Digestion

The good bacteria in your microbiome are multitaskers, especially during digestion. This bustling community of microbes works around the clock to help break down complex carbohydrates, fibers, and certain proteins that our human enzymes alone can't handle. This isn't just a small contribution; these bacteria break down food into nutrients that your body can absorb and use efficiently.

Have you ever wondered why beans are known for causing a little extra "soundtrack" in your gut? This happens because our bodies lack the enzymes needed to digest certain sugars in beans, so it's up to our gut bacteria to take over. As these bacteria break down these sugars, they produce gases like hydrogen, methane, and carbon dioxide, which, well, can make themselves known. And, while beans get a reputation for this, the same process occurs with many other types of fiber-rich foods. But what you might not realize is that, in handling these tricky foods, these microbes are doing your body a favor, contributing to a series of essential digestive processes that keep you healthy.

Breaking Down Dietary Fibers

Fiber is an essential part of a healthy diet, yet it's something that our bodies alone can't digest. Here's where your microbiome truly shines. When you consume fiber-rich foods, such as vegetables, grains, and legumes, these fibers travel largely undigested until they reach the colon, where gut bacteria go to work. These bacteria break down dietary fibers, converting them into substances called short-chain fatty acids (SCFAs), including acetate, propionate, and butyrate.

SCFAs don't just pass through your system; they serve essential functions. Butyrate, an example of SCFAs, is a primary energy source for the cells in your colon. This means your gut cells receive nourishment to stay healthy and function efficiently, thanks to your gut microbe. Butyrate also reduces inflammation, strengthens the intestinal lining, and contributes to the overall integrity of your gut barrier, which is crucial in preventing harmful substances from leaking into your bloodstream.

Assisting in Nutrient Absorption

Good bacteria in your gut play a direct role in nutrient absorption, especially when it comes to breaking down complex compounds that release essential vitamins and minerals. For instance, certain bacteria in the microbiome assist in producing and absorbing B vitamins and vitamin K, which are essential for energy production, blood clotting, and overall cellular health. By helping you absorb nutrients more effectively, your microbiome ensures that the foods you eat are converted into the vitamins and minerals your body needs to thrive.

If your microbiome is lacking diversity, your body might struggle to absorb essential nutrients, even if you're eating a nutrient-dense diet. In this way, a healthy microbiome is almost like an inner supplement, helping you access nutrients hidden within the foods you consume.

Breaking Down Protein Byproducts

While the stomach and small intestine do a lot of work breaking down proteins, some byproducts still make it to the large intestine, where the gut microbiome takes over. Certain bacteria can break down leftover protein fragments into amino acids and other beneficial compounds. This is essential, as these compounds can be repurposed within the body for energy or rebuilding tissue.

However, if there is an imbalance in your gut microbiome, it can lead to the production of less desirable byproducts, such as ammonia, which can irritate the gut lining. Having a balanced microbiome will help ensure that protein digestion continues smoothly, minimizing the risk of inflammation and digestive upset.

Regulating Gut Motility

Aside from breaking down food, your gut bacteria help control how quickly or slowly things move through your digestive system—a process known as gut motility. This is important because a very slow digestive process can lead to constipation and a buildup of toxins, while an overly fast process can result in diarrhea and nutrient loss. When your microbiome is balanced, it helps to maintain the right pace of digestion, allowing food to move through your system at an optimal rate.

One way this works is through the production of neurotransmitters, such as serotonin, by your gut bacteria. Remarkably, about 95% of the serotonin in your body is produced in the gut, where it plays a role in controlling bowel movements and the overall rhythm of digestion (Terry and Margolis, 2017).

Impact of Gut Bacteria on Immune Function

Aside from helping you break down food and extract nutrients, your gut squad plays a vital role in educating the immune system. These microbes form the front line of defense within your digestive system, working hand in hand with your immune system to identify and deal with pathological threats. Your gut squad also nourishes the gut lining and promotes the production of protective mucus. This creates a strong barrier between your gut and any harmful bacteria or viruses that might try to invade. In addition, they send signals to immune cells, regulating inflammatory responses and ensuring your body reacts appropriately when under threat. This process is essential for distinguishing between friend and foe—helping the body recognize harmful invaders while avoiding overreaction to benign or beneficial entities. This fine-tuning is particularly vital if you are living with autoimmune conditions, where the immune system mistakenly attacks your body's tissues.

A balanced composition of gut bacteria is indispensable for efficient immune function. When these microorganisms are in harmony, the immune system operates optimally, preventing inflammation that can exacerbate symptoms in Crohn's and ulcerative colitis. The presence of diverse bacterial species promotes a robust immune response, akin to having a well-trained team ready to respond to any threat efficiently. For example, certain types of beneficial bacteria, such as *Faecalibacterium spp*, produce short-chain fatty acids that nourish the cells lining your gut and strengthen your body's immune defenses. These fatty acids also help regulate inflammation, as they are a calming signal that tells your immune system when to stand down. This is particularly important in autoimmune diseases where the immune system mistakenly attacks healthy tissue, leading to chronic inflammation. The more balanced your gut bacteria, the less likely your immune system is to overreact, reducing the likelihood of flare-ups and painful symptoms. This shows how your gut microbes reduce unnecessary inflammatory signals, providing a smoother journey through chronic conditions.

Dysbiosis: An Imbalance With Consequences

When the balance of microbes in the gut is disrupted, it leads to a state known as dysbiosis. In this state, harmful bacteria often begin to outnumber the beneficial ones, throwing off the balance necessary for optimal gut health. The consequences of dysbiosis are far-reaching, impacting everything from digestive health to immune function and mental well-being. In a healthy gut, beneficial bacteria support digestion, protect against pathogens, and help maintain a strong gut barrier. When dysbiosis occurs, however, this balance collapses, resulting in increased permeability of the gut lining, also known as "leaky gut."

With a weakened gut barrier, harmful bacteria, toxins, and undigested food particles can more easily enter the bloodstream. This prompts an immune response, which may increase inflammation levels in the body. When managing inflammatory conditions like Crohn's disease or ulcerative colitis, dysbiosis can worsen symptoms, increasing the likelihood of disease flare-ups and making the gut more susceptible to infections and further imbalances. Over time, dysbiosis can contribute to chronic inflammation that impacts the gut and the entire body, making it an essential aspect of health to monitor and manage.

Consequences of Dysbiosis

Dysbiosis can result in numerous health issues, both in the short term and over an extended period. Some of the key consequences include:

Increased Inflammation and Immune Activation

When harmful bacteria overgrow or beneficial bacteria are depleted, the immune system tends to stay in a heightened state of alert. The body interprets this microbial imbalance as a potential threat, leading to increased immune activity, which in turn results in inflammation. This chronic inflammatory response can affect the gut as well as other organs, contributing to systemic inflammation and aggravating Crohn's disease and ulcerative colitis. In cases of autoimmune disease, dysbiosis may even trigger flare-ups, causing more frequent and severe symptoms.

Digestive Discomfort and Malabsorption

An imbalanced gut microbiome disrupts the efficient breakdown of foods, especially complex carbohydrates, proteins, and certain fibers. Harmful bacteria may produce gases and other byproducts that contribute to bloating, cramping, and irregular bowel movements, such as constipation or diarrhea. Over time, this microbe imbalance may impact the absorption of vital nutrients, as the necessary bacteria to help break down food and facilitate nutrient uptake may be diminished. This malabsorption can lead to nutrient deficiencies, weakening the body's defenses and exacerbating fatigue and overall discomfort in inflammatory bowel disease.

Mental Health Implications: The Gut-Brain Axis

The gut and brain are intricately connected through the gut-brain axis, a communication network that links the emotional and cognitive centers of the brain with your gut. Dysbiosis can disrupt this axis, leading to mental health implications such as anxiety, depression, and brain fog. Harmful bacteria release toxins and inflammatory compounds that can reach the brain, affecting mood and cognitive function. This can be especially challenging when you are managing Crohn's disease or ulcerative colitis, where the psychological burden of the chronic condition is already significant. Gut health, therefore, is closely tied to mental health, making dysbiosis a potential trigger for psychological stressors.

Long-Term Health Implications: Potential Link to Chronic Diseases

Chronic dysbiosis has been associated with an increased risk of various health conditions beyond the digestive tract, including cardiovascular disease, type 2 diabetes, obesity, and metabolic syndrome (Bandopadhyay and Ganguly, 2022). The persistent state of inflammation and immune activation can strain the body's systems over time, leading to long-term health complications. Managing dysbiosis becomes even more important, as it can potentially lower the risk of additional complications that would add to the challenges of IBD.

Factors That Influence Your Gut Squad Population

Research shows that low microbial diversity is linked to gastrointestinal problems like bloating and gas. When there are fewer types of bacteria, our gut struggles to manage digestion smoothly, leading to discomfort (Wei et al., 2021). Imagine preparing for a feast with only a few ingredients; the result might be less than satisfying. Similarly, a less diverse microbiome can leave us feeling bloated and uncomfortable after meals.

The following are some factors that influence your gut microbes population.

- **Diet:** What you eat is one of the most powerful influences on your microbiome. Fiber-rich foods, especially whole grains, fruits, and vegetables, act as prebiotics, feeding the beneficial bacteria in your gut. Fermented foods such as yogurt, kimchi, and sauerkraut add beneficial probiotics. In contrast, diets high in sugar and processed foods can fuel the less-friendly bacteria, leading to imbalance and possibly contributing to inflammation.

- **Antibiotic use:** While antibiotics are important in treating bacterial infections, they also impact your gut microbiome. Antibiotics don't discriminate between good and bad bacteria; they wipe out both, often leaving your gut with less diversity. After a course of antibiotics, it can take time for your microbiome to regain balance, making it especially important to consume probiotics and prebiotic-rich foods to support recovery.

- **Stress levels:** Chronic stress can affect your mental health and also influence your gut bacteria. High stress levels can disrupt the balance of your microbiome, reducing beneficial bacteria and potentially allowing harmful bacteria to grow. This disruption can lead to digestive issues and may worsen symptoms in people with inflammatory bowel diseases.

- **Exercise:** Physical activity positively impacts the diversity and health of your gut microbiome. Regular exercise encourages the growth of beneficial bacteria that produce short-chain fatty acids, which support gut health and reduce inflammation. However, balance is key; over-exercising or intense physical activity can sometimes strain the gut, especially in people with existing digestive issues.

- **Sleep quality:** Sleep plays a role in regulating your body's activities, including the gut-brain connection. Research shows that people who get adequate, high-quality sleep tend to have healthier gut bacteria, while chronic sleep deprivation is associated with a less diverse microbiome (Smith et al., 2019).

- **Hydration:** Staying well-hydrated supports digestion and helps beneficial bacteria thrive. Water assists in moving food through the digestive system, which maintains a healthy environment for gut microbes. Dehydration can slow down digestion and make the gut more susceptible to imbalances, leading to symptoms like constipation and bloating.

- **Aging:** Your microbiome changes with age. Babies have a relatively simple microbiome that becomes more diverse over time, but as we age, microbiome diversity tends to decrease. Older adults often have a less balanced microbiome, which can impact digestion and immune function. Consuming a fiber-rich diet and maintaining other healthy habits can help counteract these changes.

- **Geography and Environment:** Where you live also influences your microbiome. Different environments expose you to various bacteria, which can shape your microbiome in different ways. Rural areas tend to have more bacterial diversity due to natural surroundings, while urban environments can sometimes limit exposure to beneficial microbes.

- **Other medications:** These include proton pump inhibitors (PPIs) for acid reflux, non-steroidal anti-inflammatory drugs (NSAIDs), and even some antidepressants that can impact gut bacteria. These medications may alter pH levels or disrupt the gut lining, affecting the growth of beneficial bacteria and potentially creating an imbalance in your microbiome.

Embracing the Journey: Hope and Healing for Your Gut

Living with Crohn's disease or ulcerative colitis can feel like a constant battle, but here's the good news: You're not alone in this, and there are many ways to manage these conditions so that you can live a fulfilling, joyful life. In the coming chapters, we're diving deep into how lifestyle changes, dietary adjustments, and the smart use of medications can help keep symptoms in check, boost your quality of life, and even contribute to a healthier, more resilient gut microbiome. Think of it as building a support squad within—your "Gut Squad"—where every positive choice you make brings reinforcements to your digestive health.

Each of the strategies and insights ahead will equip you with tools to support the diversity and health of your gut bacteria, ultimately helping you feel more in control of your health journey. As we explore tips and tricks for your diet, mental health, exercise, and self-care, you'll discover how these small adjustments can bring unsatisfactory benefits, leading to a happier, healthier gut.

Fun Facts About Your Gut Bacteria

Before we get into the nitty-gritty details of managing Crohn's and colitis, let's take some time to appreciate how fascinating the gut microbiome is. Here are some fun facts about these tiny friends who play a big role in keeping you well:

- **Your microbiome is as unique as your fingerprint:** No two people have the same mix of gut bacteria. Your microbiome has developed from your birth, influenced by factors like environment, diet, and lifestyle. This uniqueness means that what works for your gut health might look a little different than what works for someone else—and that's perfectly okay! It's a reminder that personalized care is the best kind of care.

- **There are more bacteria in your gut than stars in the Milky Way:** Imagine trillions of bacteria, each with a purpose, working around the clock. There are estimated to be over 100 trillion bacteria in your gut alone—that's more than ten times the number of human cells in your body. It's truly a galaxy within you, and just like outer space, it's full of wonder and mystery.

- **Your gut bacteria can affect your mood:** Did you know that gut bacteria produce about 95% of your body's serotonin, the "feel-good" hormone? This gut-brain connection, often called the "second brain," has a big impact on how you feel. When your microbiome is balanced, it can support emotional well-being, potentially easing feelings of anxiety and depression. So, looking after your gut might just be the best kind of self-care.

- **Your microbiome changes constantly:** Unlike other parts of your body, the microbiome is not static. It shifts based on what you eat, how stressed you are, and even how much sleep you get. This means you're never too late to make a difference. With each meal, each walk outside, and each stress-relieving activity, you're actively influencing your microbiome for the better.

With all these fun facts, it's clear that your gut is an incredibly complex and intriguing system. You have the power to nurture this inner ecosystem, supporting your body in remarkable ways. The next chapter will guide you on how to make every meal an opportunity to nourish your "Gut Squad." Get ready to explore delicious ways to eat for gut health and fuel your journey to better digestion and overall wellness.

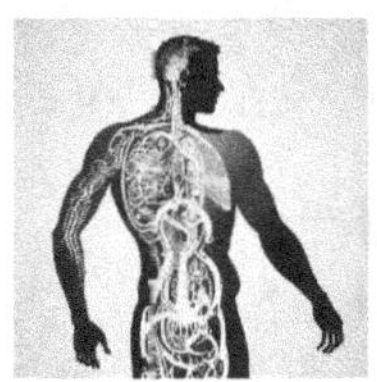

Chapter 2: Foodie Fun—Eating for Your Gut

Choosing the right foods can be a delightful adventure, especially when it involves taking care of your gut. When living with Crohn's disease or ulcerative colitis, having healthy meals holds the promise of nourishing the body and managing symptoms in a tasty way.

In this chapter, you'll journey through the various foods that boost gut health, focusing on the power of probiotics and an anti-inflammatory diet. You'll learn about the benefits of incorporating colorful fruits and vegetables, lean proteins, and healthy fats into your diet for effective symptom management. You'll also discover the advantages of fermented foods such as kimchi and tempeh, which can strengthen your digestive system. Whether you're living with an autoimmune condition or supporting someone who is, understanding these culinary options provides practical strategies for enhancing well-being. By the end of this chapter, you'll have gathered a toolbox of delicious and nutritious ways to support your gut squad, empowering you to take charge of your diet with confidence and creativity.

Probiotics and Digestive Health

Probiotics play a crucial role in maintaining digestive health, especially when managing digestive autoimmune conditions such as Crohn's disease and ulcerative colitis. Probiotics are live beneficial bacteria that support gut health by supporting the balance of the microbiome. These live beneficial microorganisms help maintain a healthy gut flora, which is essential for digestion and a robust immune system.

Recall how our gut hosts trillions of these microscopic allies, working tirelessly to break down food, absorb nutrients, and fend off harmful pathogens, and how proper functioning of these processes can make a significant difference in everyday well-being.

Incorporating probiotic-rich foods into your diet is an effective way to support gut health. Foods such as yogurt, kefir, and sauerkraut are delicious and packed with these friendly bacteria. Yogurt, for instance, contains *Lactobacillus* and *Bifidobacterium* strains known for their anti-inflammatory properties. Kefir, a fermented milk drink, offers diverse cultures that can colonize the intestinal tract better than some other probiotics. Similarly, sauerkraut, made from fermented cabbage, provides an excellent source of lactic acid bacteria—ideal companions in our quest for a balanced gut squad.

The benefits of these foods don't end with boosting the microbiome population. They can actively aid in reducing inflammation, which is a common culprit behind the uncomfortable symptoms of Crohn's and colitis. Regular consumption of these foods may lead to fewer flare-ups and more manageable day-to-day symptoms, providing you with a greater sense of control over your condition.

However, not all probiotics work uniformly for everyone. It's important to select the right strains and consume adequate amounts tailored to individual needs. For example, while *Lactobacillus rhamnosus*, found in dairy products such as yogurt and fermented foods such as kombucha or sauerkraut, has shown promise in supporting gut health for some. Others might find *Bifidobacterium infantis* more effective, which is also found in some fermented foods and supplements. The key lies in understanding your unique gut environment and consulting healthcare professionals who can provide personalized recommendations. This targeted approach ensures the probiotics you take contribute to symptom alleviation.

When dietary sources of probiotics aren't enough or feasible, probiotic supplements present a convenient alternative. Available in the form of capsules, tablets, or powders, these supplements can deliver concentrated doses of beneficial bacteria. Selecting a high-quality supplement is vital, focusing on those with scientifically validated strains and CFU counts (colony-forming units) ranging in the billions to ensure efficacy. It is usually wise to start with one prominent strain known to act against specific symptoms, then gradually incorporate additional strains based on effectiveness and tolerance. Your healthcare provider can guide you through this process.

Crafting a Balanced Anti-Inflammatory Diet

Dietary choices can be a challenging task for anyone, but it becomes even more critical and complex when managing gastrointestinal conditions. The connection between diet and inflammation is no secret; certain foods have the potential to exacerbate symptoms by triggering inflammatory responses, while others may help reduce the frequency of an inflammatory response. Through mindful selection of what goes into your meals, you can influence your gut health and alleviate some of the discomfort associated with Crohn's and ulcerative colitis.

Let's identify and understand which foods might act as triggers for inflammation. Often, processed foods, high in sugar and additives, can lead to aggravated IBD symptoms. Meanwhile, some individuals may find that dairy or gluten are common culprits. Understanding personal triggers involves a bit of self-experimentation; keeping a food diary can be an effective way to pinpoint specific items that cause flare-ups. It's this awareness and subsequent avoidance that form the foundation of managing symptoms through diet.

Once you have mapped out the foods to avoid, the next step is building a meal plan that invites anti-inflammatory benefits. A plate full of different colors with fruits and vegetables has a variety of nutrients integral to fighting inflammation. Leafy greens such as spinach and kale, alongside berries and carrots, bring vitamins, minerals, and antioxidants critical for gut health. Incorporating whole grains like quinoa and brown rice provides fiber without the irritation sometimes caused by refined grains. Lean proteins such as chicken and turkey, and plant-based options like beans play a supportive role by providing essential amino acids necessary for bodily repair and maintenance.

Healthy fats deserve a special mention, as they are potent fighters against inflammation. Sources such as avocados, nuts, and olive oil deliver monounsaturated fats, while fatty fish like salmon and sardines are rich in omega-3 fatty acids, known for their powerful anti-inflammatory properties. Including these elements in your daily meals aids in reducing inflammation and also ensures the body gets the diverse nutrients it needs to function optimally.

The inclusion of superfoods in your diet can be a delicious and natural way to reduce inflammation, particularly beneficial for individuals managing ulcerative colitis. These nutrient-packed foods provide anti-inflammatory benefits while supporting overall health. When thoughtfully integrated into your meals, they can help soothe symptoms, promote healing, and add variety to your diet. We will look into these superfoods in Chapter 8: DIY Remedies and Natural Wonders.

The Power of Mindful Eating

An often-overlooked aspect of dietary adjustments is how we consume our food. Mindful eating encapsulates the idea of being present in the moment, savoring each bite, and acknowledging the sensory experience of eating. This practice encourages slow and deliberate consumption, allowing the digestive system a better chance of processing nutrients efficiently. When you take the time to chew thoroughly and enjoy mealtimes free from distractions such as television or mobile phones, you allow your gut to work more effectively. Additionally, mindful eating often leads to greater satisfaction and a decreased likelihood of overindulgence, which can otherwise disturb the digestive balance.

Creating a supportive gut health diet doesn't need to be strictly regimented or joyless. Letting creativity flow within the confines of anti-inflammatory guidelines can yield delicious results. Explore different cuisines that naturally incorporate anti-inflammatory ingredients or experiment with fusion recipes to keep your diet interesting. Remember, incremental changes tend to be more sustainable than dramatic shifts. Start by incorporating one or two new foods or habits weekly, allowing them to become part of your lifestyle gradually rather than an overwhelming overhaul.

Communicating with healthcare professionals, such as dietitians familiar with IBD, can provide personalized clarity on food choices and nutritional needs. They can help tailor dietary plans to suit individual preferences, ensuring you don't miss out on essential nutrients while avoiding known irritants. Support networks, which may involve friends, family, or online communities, can encourage and share practical insights into the day-to-day management of Crohn's and colitis. Sharing struggles and successes with others on similar paths can offer comfort and motivation.

Fermentation and Its Benefits for Gut Health

Fermented foods are a hidden gem waiting to be explored, especially if you are focused on maintaining your gut health. Fermented foods are cherished across different cultures for their impact on gut microbiota. Let's explore further how these foods are a powerful addition to gut-friendly diets.

First off, let's demystify how fermented foods boost our gut health. The fermentation process, which involves the natural breakdown of food by microorganisms such as bacteria and yeast, increases nutrient bioavailability. This means that our bodies can extract and utilize nutrients more efficiently. Fermented foods also ramp up the production of digestive enzymes. These enzymes are crucial because they help break down foods even further, promoting better digestion and absorption. When managing Crohn's disease or ulcerative colitis, this can translate into less strain on the digestive system and potentially fewer flare-ups.

Now, you might wonder about diving into home fermentation. Fermenting your foods at home opens the door to experimenting with new flavors and textures while tailoring recipes to personal taste preferences. Imagine crafting your sauerkraut or pickles, tweaking spice levels, and discovering unique combinations that suit your palate. Such creative exploration provides enjoyment and offers valuable insights into the science behind fermentation, making it a truly educational experience.

Getting involved in community workshops or classes on fermentation can help take this journey a step further. These settings provide an opportunity to meet others interested in gut health and nutrition. Interacting with peers who share similar dietary concerns creates a supportive environment where participants can swap tips, troubleshoot issues, and learn collectively about the nutritional benefits of fermented foods. Moreover, having access to expert advice from workshop leaders or instructors can deepen understanding and inspire confidence in trying fermentation techniques at home.

Traditional foods such as yogurt, miso, or kefir might already be part of your diet, but why stop there? The world of fermentation offers a plethora of choices that are worth exploring. From tangy sauerkrauts infused with herbs to fiery kimchi rich with garlic and ginger, there's no shortage of exciting options. You may also find joy in sampling lesser-known varieties such as kvass or tepache, each offering distinct tastes and nutritional profiles.

Incorporating these fermented foods allows you to discover taste sensations you might not have encountered before. More importantly, they add meaningful diversity to your diet, which is essential for anyone conscious about gut health. Each type of food supports your body differently, providing a wide range of probiotics and nutrients beneficial to your microbiome.

Throughout this chapter, we've explored how probiotics and fermented foods can significantly maintain a balanced gut flora. With this knowledge about crafting a balanced anti-inflammatory diet, you're better equipped to make decisions that positively impact your well-being. Keep a food diary to identify triggers and embrace the vibrant variety of fruits, vegetables, whole grains, lean proteins, and healthy fats that nourish your body and soothe inflammation.

In the next chapter, we will explore how stress can trigger inflammation and exacerbate symptoms of IBD. We will also look at how you may laugh it off with some fun relaxation techniques that benefit your gut.

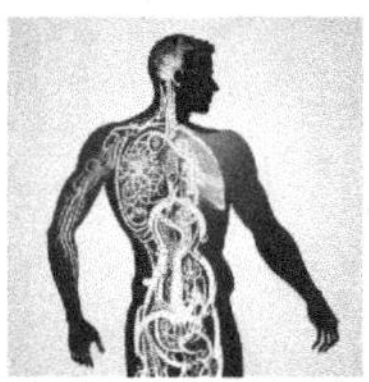

Chapter 3: The Stress Connection: Laugh It Off!

Managing stress effectively is important when living with Crohn's disease and ulcerative colitis, as these conditions can impact your emotional and physical well-being. Uncontrolled stress can exacerbate your gut symptoms and lead to increased discomfort, creating a cycle that feels difficult to break. However, exploring how laughter and humor play into stress reduction opens up new ways for coping amidst the challenges of these conditions.

In this chapter, you'll discover various mind-body techniques aimed at stress management, particularly focusing on how humor can serve as a tool for symptom reduction in Crohn's disease and ulcerative colitis.

Stress–Gut Connection

To start with, let's define stress. Stress is your body's natural reaction to a perceived threat, challenge, or pressure. It's a state of heightened alertness that prepares you to respond to danger—commonly referred to as the "fight-or-flight" response. While this response is beneficial in short bursts, chronic or long-term stress can affect your physical and mental health, especially when living with chronic conditions such as Crohn's disease or ulcerative colitis. So, what can cause stress?

Causes of Stress and Its Effects

Stress can stem from a variety of sources, and these may be different for each individual. Here are some common causes:

- **Life events:** Major life changes, such as moving, starting a new job, or dealing with a relationship challenge, can create significant stress.

- **Work pressure:** Deadlines, job security worries, or work overload can trigger high stress levels.

- **Personal relationships:** Conflicts, misunderstandings, and responsibilities in relationships, whether with family, friends, or partners, can contribute to stress.

- **Financial concerns:** Financial instability, debt, or unexpected expenses are often leading stressors.

- **Health issues:** Living with chronic conditions such as Crohn's disease and ulcerative colitis can itself be a source of stress, as can worries about flare-ups, medications, or surgeries.

- **Daily challenges:** Even everyday hassles, such as traffic, workload, or balancing responsibilities, can cause cumulative stress over time.

When you live with a chronic inflammatory condition, stress doesn't just affect your mind—it has a direct impact on your physical symptoms. Stress can lead to the following:

- **Increased inflammation:** High stress levels can worsen inflammation in the digestive tract, leading to more intense flare-ups in symptoms.

- **Digestive issues:** Common stress-induced symptoms include abdominal pain, cramping, bloating, and changes in bowel habits. For people with Crohn's or ulcerative colitis, this can mean more frequent and intense episodes of diarrhea or constipation.

- **Fatigue and low energy:** Stress can affect sleep quality and the body's energy levels, leading to chronic fatigue, which may be even more pronounced during flare-ups.

- **Appetite changes:** Stress can disrupt hunger cues, causing overeating, undereating, or simply disrupting digestion in a way that leads to discomfort.

- **Mood changes:** Anxiety, irritability, and even depression are common symptoms linked to chronic stress, and these can further exacerbate symptoms by impacting hormone levels and immune function.

How Stress Exacerbates Symptoms in Crohn's Disease and Ulcerative Colitis

Stress influences the body in different ways, impacting everything from hormone levels to immune function. When you are under stress, the body releases stress hormones like cortisol and adrenaline. These hormones prompt the immune system to produce inflammatory cytokines, which are chemical messengers that signal inflammation in the body. This worsens conditions already marked by chronic inflammation, such as IBD, which can make symptoms significantly worse, leading to flare-ups.

Gut motility can be affected by stress, disrupting the gut-brain axis—the essential communication network between your digestive system and brain. Stress hormones can either slow down or speed up the digestive process, leading to symptoms such as cramping, diarrhea, or constipation. These symptoms become difficult to handle when you are living with IBD.

Chronic stress also alters the balance of bacteria in the gut microbiome. When stress is prolonged, beneficial bacteria in the gut are reduced, while harmful bacteria can thrive. This microbial imbalance tends to escalate inflammation and prompts a heightened immune response, worsening IBD symptoms and making them harder to control.

Another effect of stress is its weakening of the gut barrier, which regulates what passes from the digestive tract into the bloodstream. Under sustained pressure, the gut lining can become compromised, resulting in what's known as "leaky gut" or increased intestinal permeability. When this barrier becomes weak, harmful substances more easily enter the bloodstream, triggering immune responses and inflammation that aggravate symptoms in Crohn's disease and ulcerative colitis.

Stress Reduction Through Mind–Body Practices

Now that you know how stress can affect you, harnessing effective mind-body practices can be a game-changer in managing stress and enhancing gut health. Let's look into some stress reduction practices and how they bring distinct benefits, aiding your mental clarity and physical well-being. Let's delve into some of these practices and how they foster improved health.

Mindfulness Meditation

Mindfulness meditation is a powerful tool that cultivates present-moment awareness. When you consistently practice mindfulness, you become more attuned to your thoughts and feelings, allowing you to recognize stress triggers early on. This heightened awareness acts as a buffer against anxiety, providing a sense of control over your emotional responses. When you are dealing with the daily unpredictability of ulcerative colitis, you might find solace in knowing that you can acknowledge your stress without letting it dominate your day. To get started with mindfulness, set aside a few quiet minutes each day, focus on your breath, and gently guide your mind back to your normal self whenever it begins to wander. This simple practice can gradually build resilience against stress, creating space for a calmer, more balanced life.

Breathwork

Breathwork techniques are a simple yet powerful tool to help you manage stress and support your well-being. These intentional breathing practices go beyond the automatic breaths you take every day. By focusing on your breathing, you can create a calming effect on your mind and body, reduce tension, and navigate challenging moments with greater ease. Let's break down how breathwork works and how you can use it effectively, even in the middle of a busy day or during a flare-up of symptoms.

The science behind breathwork is that it increases oxygen flow to the body, which helps regulate the nervous system. When you're stressed, your body often shifts into "fight or flight" mode, causing shallow, rapid breathing. This can make you feel even more anxious. Intentional breathing, on the other hand, encourages your body to switch to "rest and digest" mode, which calms the mind, relaxes the muscles, and slows the heart rate. Think of breathwork as your body's natural reset button, available anytime you need it. Let's briefly look into some types of breathwork.

Diaphragmatic Breathing

Diaphragmatic breathing, also known as belly breathing, focuses on engaging the diaphragm, a large muscle located below your lungs. This technique can help you breathe more deeply and efficiently, allowing for a greater intake of oxygen. Here's how you can practice diaphragmatic breathing:

1. **Find a comfortable position:** Sit in a chair with your feet flat on the ground, or lie down on your back. Place one hand on your chest and the other on your belly.

2. **Inhale deeply through your nose:** Focus on filling your belly with air. You should feel the hand on your belly rise, while the hand on your chest remains still.

3. **Exhale slowly through your mouth:** Let the air escape fully, feeling your belly fall as you release the breath.

4. **Repeat:** Continue this cycle for 5–10 minutes, paying attention to the rhythm of your breath.

This simple practice can be done anywhere—whether you're at home, in a meeting, or stuck in traffic. It helps ground you and reduce feelings of overwhelm.

4-7-8 Method

The 4-7-8 breathing technique is another highly effective method to calm your mind and body, especially during moments of acute stress or when you're preparing for bed. It's a structured breathing pattern that helps slow your heart rate and promotes relaxation. Here's how it works:

1. **Inhale:** Close your mouth and inhale quietly through your nose for a count of 4.

2. **Hold your breath:** Hold the breath for a count of 7. This allows oxygen to circulate throughout your body.

3. **Exhale:** Open your mouth slightly and exhale completely through your mouth for a count of 8, making a whooshing sound as you do so.

4. **Repeat:** Perform this cycle 4 times, or until you feel calmer.

This technique works wonders in high-pressure situations, such as a social gathering where you feel uneasy or during a flare-up of symptoms. It's discreet and can be done without anyone noticing, making it a convenient tool to have in your stress-management toolbox.

Yoga

Yoga is more than just a form of exercise; it's a holistic practice that nurtures physical and emotional well-being, offering notable benefits for gut health. Through enhancing blood flow, reducing stress, and promoting body awareness, yoga directly influences your digestive system and overall wellness.

Specific yoga poses stimulate the digestive organs, facilitating smoother digestion and alleviating discomforts like bloating or constipation. Additionally, yoga's emphasis on mindful breathing and gentle movement helps relax the nervous system, counteracting stress—a major trigger for digestive issues.

Let's have a breakdown of beginner-friendly yoga poses that can support digestion and reduce stress:

Cat-Cow Pose (Marjaryasana-Bitilasana)

You can perform the cat-cow pose by following the steps below.

- **Step 1:** Start with your hands and knees in a tabletop position, with your wrists directly under your shoulders and knees under your hips.

- **Step 2:** Inhale deeply as you arch your back, dropping your belly toward the floor and lifting your head and tailbone (Cow Pose).

- **Step 3:** Exhale fully as you round your back, tucking your chin to your chest and pulling your belly toward your spine (Cat Pose).

- **Step 4:** Repeat this flow for 5–10 breaths, moving at your own pace.

This exercise helps to stimulate the abdominal muscles, massages the intestines, and enhances spinal flexibility.

Child's Pose (Balasana)

Another simple yoga pose you can try at home is the child's pose. The steps are below.

- **Step 1:** Kneel on the floor with your big toes touching and knees spread apart.

- **Step 2:** Lower your torso between your thighs, stretching your arms forward or resting them alongside your body.

- **Step 3:** Rest your forehead on the ground and breathe deeply for 1–2 minutes.

This activity helps relax the lower back and abdomen while promoting calmness and easing digestive tension.

If you're new to yoga or have limited mobility, gentle forms like restorative yoga or chair yoga provide an accessible starting point. These approaches prioritize comfort and can be just as effective for improving gut health.

Progressive Muscle Relaxation (PMR)

PMR is a technique that involves systematically tensing and then relaxing various muscle groups. This method helps you identify physical manifestations of stress, empowering you to consciously release tension. Its beauty lies in its simplicity and versatility—once learned, PMR can be practiced almost anywhere, whether you're sitting at your desk or lying in bed. You can start by taking a comfortable position, then focus on one muscle group at a time, such as your shoulders or calves. Tense the muscles for a few seconds, then slowly release, noticing the sensation of relaxation washing over you. With regular practice, PMR can become an intuitive habit that leads to reductions in physical stress symptoms, contributing to overall comfort and ease.

Integrating these mind-body practices into daily life requires commitment but promises rewarding outcomes. They serve as proactive measures that support symptom management and also enhance the quality of life. Cultivating these habits can lead to a harmonious relationship with your body, transforming stress from a daunting adversary into a manageable part of life.

Humor for Your Emotional Well-Being

Humor plays a crucial role in managing the day-to-day challenges of living with chronic medical conditions. Most chronic diseases aren't just physically demanding; they also place a heavy emotional burden on you and your support networks. Finding light amid these ongoing struggles isn't just about delivering momentary relief; it can influence one's physical health positively.

Laughter therapy, for example, has been shown to lower stress hormones such as cortisol and adrenaline (Akimbekov and Razzaque, 2021). Recall how when we are stressed, our bodies enter a flight-or-fight mode, which amplifies inflammation—something that is harmful when dealing with autoimmune diseases. Participating in laughter therapy doesn't mean you're ignoring your condition; instead, it's a way to create a positive atmosphere that fosters connections with others. Imagine attending a laughter yoga session where the room is filled with joyful sounds, allowing participants to feel less isolated and more supported. The shared experience of laughing can help bridge gaps, offering an emotional release that is nurturing and healing.

Comedy Content

Aside from structured sessions, finding comedy content through films, books, or stand-up routines can further release some stress. Watching a funny movie or TV series invites everyone around to share in the humor. This communal form of entertainment encourages sharing outside the screen too. Swapping favorite jokes or scenes improves bonding with family, friends, or even support groups. Engaging in these activities builds supportive bonds rooted in mutual enjoyment and understanding. Moreover, it promotes self-compassion by allowing you to view yourself and your life with a lighter perspective, taking the sting out of everyday frustrations.

A practical guideline to share or enjoy humor in daily life can involve setting up a weekly family night featuring comedy shows or movies. Sharing such experiences strengthens family ties and positions humor as a habitual part of life, fostering an environment ripe with support and comfort.

Journaling

Humor journaling serves as another interesting approach, shifting focus from struggles to positives. Chronicling daily experiences with humor demands a conscious effort to find levity in ordinary moments. It's a personal exercise that encourages writers to reflect on their day, noting down incidents that sparked laughter or amusement. Over time, keeping such a journal enhances resilience and serves as a record of personal triumphs. You will get the chance to reflect on your growth, recognizing how far you've come by concentrating on moments of joy rather than pain.

When starting a humor journal, begin with short, weekly reflections. Highlight amusing occurrences or funny mishaps, and revisit them periodically to appreciate personal progress and maintain a lighter outlook on life.

The power of humor extends well beyond momentary distraction; it represents a vital tool in coping with the emotional challenges of chronic illness. While these practices won't cure physical ailments, they can improve the overall quality of life by promoting emotional wellness, strengthening relationships, and cultivating resilience.

Emotional Resilience Techniques

In the face of chronic medical conditions such as Crohn's disease and ulcerative colitis, emotional resilience can be a powerful ally. Living with a chronic condition often leads to feelings of isolation, but nurturing relationships with family, friends, or support groups offers a vital sense of community. For those experiencing these health challenges, such connections provide a space for shared experiences, creating an empowering environment where you realize you are not alone in your journey. Group gatherings, whether in-person or virtual, can create intimacy and understanding, enabling emotional exchanges that lighten individual burdens.

Social support networks do more than offer emotional comfort; they can also play a role in symptom management. When people share their stories, insights, and coping mechanisms, it helps encourage others to explore new ways to handle their conditions. These shared moments ignite hope and inspire action, prompting individuals to try different approaches for stress reduction or lifestyle adjustments. For caregivers and family members, participating actively in these communities opens opportunities to understand their loved one's experiences, deepening empathy and reinforcing supportive bonds.

Another powerful tool for building emotional resilience is cognitive reframing. This technique involves shifting one's perspective to view situations from a different angle. It's about challenging negative thought patterns and replacing them with more constructive interpretations. When it comes to chronic medical conditions, cognitive reframing might mean acknowledging the difficulties but choosing to focus on personal strengths and small victories. By altering your mindset, you can alleviate psychological burdens, reducing stress and anxiety.

In practice, instead of focusing solely on the limitations posed by your condition, you might embrace moments of progress, no matter how small. A day without pain, a fruitful doctor's appointment, or completing a task despite fatigue can all serve as reminders of resilience and capability. Health professionals can introduce exercises in cognitive reframing, guiding you to identify and challenge unhelpful thoughts.

Practicing gratitude is another key element in fostering emotional resilience. Gratitude doesn't diminish the reality of living with a chronic illness but emphasizes focusing attention on what's working well despite ongoing challenges. Regularly reflecting on things to be thankful for can transform perspectives, engendering positivity and helping to cultivate an optimistic outlook. Whether it's appreciation for a supportive partner, access to quality healthcare, or simply the beauty of a sunrise, focusing on gratitude nurtures mindfulness and contentment.

Creativity also provides another robust avenue for emotional expression and resilience. Engaging in creative outlets—such as painting, writing, music, or any form of self-expression—offers a constructive way to process emotions and release stress. Creative activities allow you to escape into a world of imagination and possibility, providing both pleasure and a sense of accomplishment. This process can enhance emotional well-being by offering a break from the realities of illness, allowing space for joy and relaxation.

You can explore various forms of creativity that resonate best with you, whether it's through art, dance, or cooking. Caregivers and family members can support this exploration by engaging in creative activities together, fostering stronger bonds and mutual enjoyment.

The interplay between social connection, cognitive reframing, gratitude, and creative expression creates a comprehensive framework for managing emotional challenges associated with chronic illnesses. Each strategy supports and enhances the other, contributing to a resilient mindset that embraces both struggles and triumphs.

In this chapter, we've explored the vital connection between stress management and symptom reduction for those living with Crohn's disease and ulcerative colitis. By incorporating mind-body techniques such as mindfulness meditation, yoga, progressive muscle relaxation, and humor into daily routines, you can gain control over your stress levels, which play a significant role in managing chronic conditions.

In the next chapter, we will explore how exercise can help improve your digestion and digestive symptoms and what kind of exercises you can try. See you there.

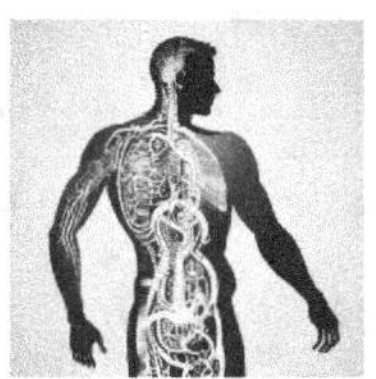

Chapter 4: Exercise With a Smile—Move Your Gut!

"Exercise with a smile" is about finding joy in movement while reaping the benefits it offers. The intertwined relationship between physical activity and gut health provides a roadmap to improving digestive well-being through enjoyable practices. This chapter invites you to explore how integrating exercise into daily routines can transform your relationship with your body, enhancing your physical health and boosting mental well-being by reducing stress.

As we break down these techniques, you'll learn how small adjustments can yield significant rewards for gut health, underscoring the importance of consistency and enjoyment in your fitness journey. Let's begin.

Exercises That Enhance Gut Motility

In this section, we will look into exercises that help improve gut motility, aid digestion, and ease daily symptoms. I've included a variety of exercises here to suit different preferences. As a fitness class instructor, I encourage you to try various classes, hit the gym, and explore different sports. Don't let your condition hold you back from doing what you love—I'm still able to lift weights, run, and even tackle burpees with my colitis affecting me!

I also have a dog, Dennis, a Wire Fox Terrier, who has provided me with invaluable support, both mentally and physically. I wouldn't be without him. As an author, I've even written a book about his adventures, *The Adventures of Dennis the Wire Fox Terrier: The Enchanted Forest—A Fantasy Fairytale*, available on Amazon.

Yoga

We looked into yoga on stress reduction techniques, but there is more than one advantage to yoga. Gentle yoga is an excellent foundation for improving gut motility and overall digestive health. This form of exercise involves a variety of poses that can facilitate the massaging of the intestines, thereby stimulating digestion. Poses such as the supine twist or seated forward bend are particularly effective in gently compressing and decompressing the abdominal region, promoting movement through the digestive tract. These poses help in moving digestive content and also enhance blood flow to the digestive organs, providing them with the nutrients and oxygen they need to function efficiently. These exercises may help you find relief from symptoms such as bloating and constipation.

Walking

Stepping outside for a brisk walk or indulging in light aerobics can improve gut health by expediting intestinal transit time. As you move, your circulation increases, supplying blood more rapidly to your gut, which enhances its overall functionality. This type of exercise doesn't just get the heart pumping—it aids your entire body systems to improve their optimal functioning.

Walking provides a low-impact option perfect for anyone, regardless of fitness level or experience. Imagine walking through a park, surrounded by nature, embracing each step with intention. The simplicity of this act itself holds transformative potential, encouraging engagement with one's environment and offering moments of peaceful reflection. Similarly, light aerobics at home or in a community setting serve as a wonderful way to elevate mood while simultaneously supporting digestive processes.

Core Strengthening Exercises

The core includes deep muscles such as the diaphragm, pelvic floor, and transverse abdominis—all key players in maintaining digestive health. Exercises such as planks, bridges, or gentle Pilates can strengthen these muscles, providing stability to the midsection. With a strong core, there is less pressure on the digestive system, allowing it to function without unnecessary constraints or blockages.

Building a stronger core is about foundational support, physically and metaphorically. A robust core means better posture, improved balance, and reduced back pain. The confidence you will gain from knowing that your body can support you through diverse activities can encourage a more active lifestyle, pivotal for ongoing disease management.

Dance and Zumba

Dance and Zumba offer a unique blend of exercise and enjoyment that can do wonders for gut health. Through rhythmic movements that engage multiple muscle groups, dance becomes a dynamic workout that reduces stress while improving your coordination and cardiovascular health. When you dance, whether it's salsa, hip-hop, or simply swaying to your favorite tunes, you're partaking in an energetic activity that elevates mood, encourages social interaction, and creates a sense of community.

Zumba classes, in particular, blend various musical styles with aerobic routines, creating a fun yet beneficial experience that engages your mind and body. These classes provide a space where participants feel encouraged and supported within a group setting while working toward individual health goals.

Adapting Physical Activity to Energy Levels

Understanding how to balance exercise with personal energy levels and symptoms is crucial when managing Crohn's disease and ulcerative colitis. When starting, it can be challenging, but making exercise a part of your daily life can boost your gut health while helping you manage and cope with the symptoms.

One fundamental strategy is listening to your body. It's important to recognize when you're feeling good and can push yourself a bit more or when it's time to rest. This self-awareness can prevent unnecessary strain, especially during flare-ups. Everyone's body has different signals, so learning yours can help you become your best advocate.

Rest days aren't just a luxury—they're a necessity. They allow your body to heal and recuperate, which is particularly important if you're experiencing symptoms. But this doesn't mean you should be completely inactive. Light activities, such as slow walks or restorative yoga, offer gentle movement that keeps your body in motion without overexerting it. These activities can also serve as a mental break, providing a moment of peace and relaxation that might ease the stress affecting your gut.

Shorter, more frequent workouts are another great strategy. Instead of pushing through an hour-long workout, breaking it into 10- or 15-minute sessions throughout the day can make fitness more manageable. This approach adapts to your energy levels and offers flexibility. Perhaps a short morning walk before breakfast, followed by some stretching or light strength training in the afternoon, can have substantial health benefits over time. As a bonus, shorter sessions can fit seamlessly into busy schedules, making it easier to stay consistent, even when you're not feeling your best.

Another key aspect of maintaining a regular exercise routine is finding activities you enjoy. This isn't just about staying active; it's about creating a lifestyle that is rewarding and sustainable. Whether it's dancing, swimming, or hiking, engaging in activities that bring joy will encourage continuity and exploration. Over time, they become more than mere exercises—they evolve into hobbies. Enjoyable exercises foster motivation and can lead to building a community around shared interests. Participating in group classes or clubs allows you to share experiences with others, offering both social connection and potential emotional support, which can be incredibly valuable in managing chronic conditions.

While these approaches offer pathways to integrating exercise into life with Crohn's or ulcerative colitis, everyone's journey is distinct. Finding what works best may require experimentation with different activities, schedules, or intensities. It's important to remember that progress isn't always linear. There will be good days and bad days—embracing this fluctuation allows for a realistic understanding of your body's needs.

Linking Exercise and Gut Health

Engaging in consistent exercise helps lower levels of inflammatory markers in the body, contributing to more effective management of autoimmune disorders. This may be through aerobic exercises such as cycling or swimming, or strength training with weights. Including movement in daily routines plays an indispensable role in soothing the gut.

Beyond inflammation control, exercise contributes to maintaining a balanced microbiome. Remember how the gut microbiome consists of trillions of bacteria that reside in our intestines and are crucial for digestion and nutrient absorption? Regular movement can positively influence the diversity and health of this microbial community. Exercise encourages the growth of beneficial bacteria while curbing the number of harmful strains.

This balance supports optimal digestive function and maximizes nutrient uptake, both essential when grappling with digestive diseases.

Living with Crohn's disease and ulcerative colitis can trigger stress and anxiety, given the unpredictability of flare-ups and the need for constant management. However, exercise is a proven strategy to combat stress, releasing endorphins—often called "feel-good" hormones—that boost mood and reduce anxiety. Activities such as yoga or tai chi, which emphasize mindfulness and deep breathing, can be particularly effective. When stress levels decrease, there is less likelihood of triggering gut-related issues, creating a positive feedback loop that enhances your overall well-being.

Having a regular exercise routine is not solely about immediate relief but encourages lasting lifestyle changes that benefit gut health in the long run. Over time, these small yet significant efforts compound, leading to improved digestion, better energy levels, and enhanced resilience against disease.

As with any health strategy, personalization matters. You should tailor your exercise plans to suit personal preferences, energy levels, and symptom severity. Consulting healthcare providers or fitness professionals can ensure that your exercise program is safe, effective, and aligned with your health goals.

As you explore what feels best, remember that every step taken is a push toward improved gut health and a more empowered you. In the next chapter, we will look into the different medication options available to help control symptoms of Crohn's disease and ulcerative colitis.

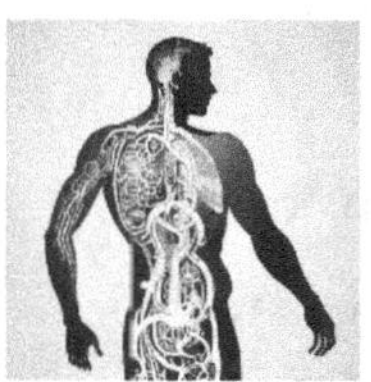

Chapter 5: Medication Mingle—Finding Your Perfect Match

Finding the right medication for Crohn's disease and ulcerative colitis can feel like a never-ending quest, where each option carries its potential to ease symptoms and improve daily life. The journey toward finding your perfect match is rooted in the science of medicine and also in the art of personal alignment—identifying what works best for you amidst the myriad choices. While this path may be challenging, I want you to know that you are not alone; many have trodden these halls, learning through experiences that are personal and shared. It's a process that involves more than selecting a pill from a bottle; it's an ongoing dialogue between you and those dedicated to your wellness, ensuring each step feels as if it's finely attuned to your needs and lifestyle. I've had to try various medications to find the right balance to keep my colitis in check. For some, the first medication may be the right fit, which is great, but for others, it might be a journey to find a regimen that brings relief. In some cases, it may even lead to surgery. Rest assured, though, that your clinical team has your best interests at heart and is working to find the best possible outcome for you.

This chapter delves into the landscape of medication options available for managing Crohn's disease and ulcerative colitis, offering insights into how various treatments function and their intended roles in symptom management.

Overview of Medication Options

Understanding the available medications is a critical step toward managing autoimmune conditions such as ulcerative colitis and Crohn's disease effectively. Let's explore some common medications that play key roles in treating these autoimmune diseases.

Biologics

Biologics are often heralded as game-changers in autoimmune disorders. These medications are derived from living organisms and work by targeting specific components of the immune system. For many people, biologics help maintain remission, reducing inflammation and allowing the intestines to heal over time. Drugs like vedolizumab, infliximab, adalimumab, and ustekinumab belong to this category. They are usually administered through infusions or injections.

The primary advantage of biologics lies in their ability to offer long-term control over symptoms when other treatment methods have failed. You must work closely with your healthcare providers to monitor the effectiveness and any potential side effects of these treatments. This collaboration ensures that the chosen biologic continues to be the right fit for your health needs.

Aminosalicylates

Commonly referred to as 5-ASAs, these provide a layer of defense against the symptoms of Crohn's disease and ulcerative colitis. These drugs primarily focus on reducing inflammation directly in the intestinal lining. Medications such as mesalamine, sulfasalazine, and balsalazide fall into this category and are generally prescribed for mild to moderate cases of these conditions. Unlike some other treatments, aminosalicylates tend to have fewer systemic effects since they concentrate their action locally within the gut. Most people often find them beneficial for maintaining remission of ulcerative colitis, helping to alleviate symptoms such as diarrhea and abdominal pain. As with any medication, it's important to adhere to their dosing schedules and communicate with your doctors about how well these medications are managing your symptoms.

Corticosteroids

In contrast, corticosteroids serve as a more immediate response to flare-ups, providing powerful anti-inflammatory effects that can rapidly ease severe symptoms. Commonly used corticosteroids include prednisone and budesonide. These work by suppressing overall immune activity for immediate reduction of inflammation. While corticosteroids can be incredibly effective in the short term, they are typically not suitable for long-term use due to their potential to cause significant side effects. These may include weight gain, osteoporosis, high blood pressure, and increased susceptibility to infections. Therefore, you and your healthcare providers need to discuss the risks and benefits thoroughly before embarking on a corticosteroid regimen. Short-term use, combined with a clear plan for tapering off the medication, helps minimize these risks while controlling acute disease flares.

Immunomodulators

If you do not respond adequately to first-line treatments, immunomodulators offer another therapeutic avenue. These medications work by dampening the body's immune response, helping to prevent ongoing attacks on the gastrointestinal tract. Azathioprine, mercaptopurine, and methotrexate are examples of immunomodulators that are effectively used to control symptoms of autoimmune diseases. It can take weeks or even months for these drugs to reach their full effect, so patience and consistent monitoring are essential during this period. Although immunomodulators can result in notable improvements in condition management, they also require careful attention due to potential side effects such as an increased risk of infections or liver complications. Regular blood tests are often recommended to ensure safe and effective use of these agents.

Discussing Side Effects With Health Professionals

Communication with healthcare providers is essential when dealing with any chronic condition. Recognizing typical reactions to medications can help you engage in proactive dialogues with your doctors. Common side effects might range from mild symptoms such as headaches or nausea to more serious issues like liver problems or infections. When you get familiar with these potential outcomes, you can be better prepared to communicate any experienced side effects and work collaboratively with your healthcare team to address concerns immediately.

You should feel encouraged to ask questions and be honest about your experiences. This will create a collaborative approach that benefits both you and your health provider. Before appointments, it helps to jot down any specific questions or concerns, no matter how trivial they might seem. For example, consider asking: "Are these side effects normal?", "What should I do if they worsen?", or "Are there any signs I should look out for that might indicate a serious problem?" These questions can guide discussions and ensure that you receive valuable feedback.

If you are finding your current medications unsatisfactory, exploring alternative treatments can offer significant reassurance under the guidance of your doctor. It's important to know that switching medications isn't a setback; instead, it can be a strategic step toward improved health outcomes. New medications may present different side effect profiles, which can sometimes align better with your needs and lifestyle. Open conversations with healthcare providers about all available options can help ensure that treatment adjustments are made based on informed decisions. Your healthcare team often has experience with various medications and can suggest alternatives that might fit better with the patient's unique circumstances.

Tracking side effects through a medication journal is another powerful tool you can use in your favor. By keeping detailed records of any adverse effects, you can establish patterns over time. This practice aids in personal awareness and also provides concrete data to discuss with doctors. Recording details such as the date, time, nature, and intensity of side effects, along with any relevant activities or dietary changes, can unveil correlations that might otherwise be missed. For instance, if certain side effects consistently appear after meals, this could lead to discussions about diet adjustments or meal timing modifications.

When preparing questions in advance and maintaining open lines of communication, you position yourself as an active partner in your healthcare, creating stronger relationships with your providers. This partnership enables personalized treatment plans tailored to meet individual needs, ultimately improving wellness outcomes.

When faced with options, such as exploring alternative medications, it's pivotal to maintain an open mind and trust in the process. Each individual's response to medication is unique, making it crucial to exchange regular updates and insights with healthcare professionals.

Tracking Medication Effectiveness Over Time

When embarking on any treatment plan, establishing baseline health measures is essential. This foundational step lays the groundwork for assessing how your body responds over time. Baselines might include factors such as weight, blood pressure, inflammatory markers in the blood, and even mental health indicators. When you have an accurate picture of your pre-treatment state, you can more easily pinpoint changes, whether positive or negative, that occur after starting a new medication. Think of it as creating a roadmap; without knowing where you started, it's challenging to appreciate how far you've come. Always keep close communication with your medical team. Many hospitals offer support lines, often with a nurse available to consult if you experience any change in symptoms. I regularly submit a stool sample to check my calprotectin levels, which helps monitor inflammation in my gut and indicates whether my condition is under control.

Once a baseline is established, a practical tool at your disposal is maintaining a symptom diary. This simple method involves daily entries documenting how you feel, noting specific symptoms, their intensity, and frequency. Include details like diet, stress levels, and sleep quality, which can all influence your condition. With regular entries, patterns begin to emerge, helping you understand triggers or improvements linked to your medication regimen.

Try setting a specific time each day to make your entry, perhaps alongside another routine activity such as morning coffee or bedtime reading. The beauty of a symptom diary lies in its simple yet profound ability to reveal insights into your treatment journey. While this process may seem tedious at first, the benefits are substantial—offering you a clear narrative of your health story and an invaluable tool for discussions with healthcare providers.

Your doctor will evaluate clinical data alongside your observations, making adjustments to your treatment plan as necessary. Perhaps a dosage tweak is needed, or maybe an entirely different medication would be more effective.

Flexibility is another important consideration as you evaluate progress. Just because a medication is initially prescribed doesn't mean it's set in stone forever. Treatment plans should evolve based on their outcomes. If persistent symptoms continue to disrupt your life or if side effects become intolerable, it may be time to reevaluate. Embracing a flexible mindset allows you to engage proactively with your healthcare team, exploring alternative approaches when the current regimen doesn't meet expectations. Remember, medication management is a dynamic process tailored to fit your unique needs over time.

In this ongoing evaluation, there are several focus areas to consider. One is the tangible improvement of symptoms—are you experiencing fewer flare-ups or less severe pain? But also think about quality-of-life enhancements. Can you partake in activities previously hindered by your condition? Are you enjoying better mental health due to reduced anxiety over symptom management? Such qualitative changes, while harder to quantify, are equally significant in measuring success.

Additionally, listening to your body plays a vital role. Your instinctive sense of wellness is a powerful indicator. Perhaps a particular medication makes you feel fundamentally "off," even if objective markers say otherwise. Don't discount these gut feelings; discuss them with your healthcare provider, who can help decipher whether changes in your treatment plan might be warranted.

To further enrich this process, consider collaborating closely with caregivers or family members. Their observations offer another perspective on your health journey. They might notice mood changes or energy fluctuations that align with your medication record, offering additional data points. Open communication with those who support you enhances overall understanding, fostering a collaborative environment conducive to effective medication management.

In this chapter, we have looked at the different types of medications used in managing Crohn's disease and ulcerative colitis. We have also looked into the importance of close collaboration with healthcare providers, helping you make informed decisions that align with your personal health goals. We have also explored how engaging in open dialogues with doctors helps manage symptoms effectively and empowers you to take charge of your health journeys. Managing chronic conditions requires a combination of medical and holistic management; in the next chapter, we will explore the power of positivity and how your mindset can affect your health. See you in the next chapter as we embrace positivity over negativity.

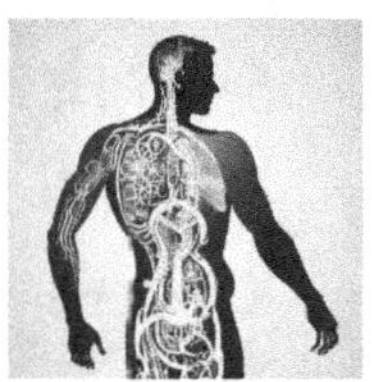

Chapter 6: The Power of Positivity—Mind Over Matter

Positivity holds a remarkable power in shaping our lives, especially when living with a chronic condition. Harnessing this power involves embracing strategies that foster a positive outlook, which can significantly impact daily management, symptom perception, and overall health outcomes.

In this chapter, we will delve into practical mindset strategies designed to improve positivity and health outcomes for anyone living with Crohn's and ulcerative colitis. This approach has truly helped me cultivate a positive mindset, empowering me to overcome obstacles along the way. I'm confident it will be just as beneficial for you.

Developing a Gratitude Practice

When we consider the role of gratitude in managing chronic conditions such as Crohn's disease and ulcerative colitis, it's not just about a fleeting moment of thankfulness; it becomes a powerful tool for improving mental well-being. Gratitude is more than a moment of feeling thankful; it involves acknowledging its psychological benefits. Research suggests that individuals who practice gratitude experience reduced stress and anxiety levels (Fekete and Deichert, 2022). This happens because focusing on positive aspects creates an emotional buffer against life's challenges. This positivity can translate into noticeable differences in symptom perception and coping abilities. Let's look into some ways you may develop gratitude.

Gratitude Journey

One of the ways to cultivate gratitude is through having a gratitude journal. This simple yet impactful activity involves writing down positive moments or things you are thankful for each day. Reflecting on these entries helps shift attention toward what is appreciated rather than dwelling on difficulties. Over time, this reinforces a more positive mindset. You can revisit your journals during tough times; this will remind you of good experiences and nurture resilience. It's akin to planting seeds of positivity; with consistent care, they grow and flourish, offering comfort and perspective when needed most.

Express Your Gratitude With Others

Sharing gratitude with others can enhance your social connections. Expressing gratitude to family, friends, or caregivers strengthens relationships by showing appreciation for their presence and support. This gesture strengthens your support network, which is vital when managing a chronic condition. When gratitude is shared, it invites openness and compassion, creating an environment where mutual understanding thrives. Stronger relationships provide a safety net, offering emotional and practical support that can ease the burdens of daily management.

To make gratitude a lasting habit, consistency is key. You can be consistent by setting reminders to write or finding ways to integrate gratitude into routine activities. For example, pairing gratitude reflections with morning tea or evening wind-down routines makes it easier to remember and makes journaling part of your day. Technology can also be of use, as some apps are designed for gratitude journaling and offer prompts and notifications.

The idea is to weave gratitude seamlessly into everyday activities, allowing it to naturally influence your thoughts and behaviors. As this habit takes root, it enhances mental flexibility and adaptability—qualities essential for managing chronic conditions effectively.

Examples Of Gratitude Messages

If you have no idea where to start with gratitude messages, below are some examples.

Gratitude Message for Others

- "Thank you for always being there when I need support; your kindness and understanding have truly been a gift in my life."

- "I'm so grateful for your presence and encouragement. You bring so much positivity and light, and I couldn't ask for a better friend."

- "I truly appreciate all the ways you've helped me grow. Your advice, patience, and wisdom have made an incredible impact on my journey."

- "Words can't express how grateful I am for your generosity. Your selflessness and thoughtfulness mean the world to me."

- "Thank you for the countless ways you show up for me. I'm blessed to have someone so reliable and caring in my life."

Gratitude Messages for Self

- "I'm grateful for my strength and perseverance. Living with a chronic condition isn't easy, but each day I wake up determined to keep going, showing myself the compassion I deserve."

- "Thank you, self, for staying patient on the tough days. My journey hasn't been straightforward, but I'm proud of how I keep pushing forward with resilience and hope."

- "I appreciate my body for carrying me through, even when it feels like a struggle. I'm learning to honor every small victory and remind myself that I am stronger than I may feel."

- "I'm grateful for the kindness I show myself on the days when symptoms are hard to manage. Living with this condition has taught me patience and how to celebrate small steps."

Positivity in Affirmation

Affirmation is another underestimated tool for building a positive mindset, especially when facing life's challenges. Unlike gratitude, which focuses on appreciating things as they are, affirmation centers on intentionally speaking positive beliefs into your life to shift your focus toward hope and self-worth. While gratitude celebrates what you have, affirmation encourages you to believe in what you can become and achieve. This makes it a great technique for anyone managing a chronic condition, as it empowers you to see beyond immediate struggles and focus on the possibilities for strength and growth.

Living with a chronic condition can often lead to feelings of frustration, self-doubt, or limitation. In times like these, affirmations work as grounding statements to counter negative thoughts and provide reassurance.

When practiced consistently, you can improve your mental resilience and help you respond to difficult days with more self-compassion and patience. When you affirm what you want to feel or believe, you're actively choosing to focus on your potential rather than your limitations, creating a mindset that can handle the ups and downs smoothly. Even when symptoms are challenging, positive affirmations can remind you of your ability to endure and adapt, helping you build a strong inner voice that cheers you on, no matter what.

Fun Affirmations and Visualization Exercises

Incorporating affirmations into your daily life can be a refreshing ritual, and adding visualization exercises can make them even more powerful. Here are a few fun affirmations and visualizations to get you started:

"I am strong and resilient."

Close your eyes and picture yourself as a mighty tree with deep roots extending into the earth, keeping you steady no matter what winds blow. Visualize yourself standing tall and unwavering, feeling a strong connection to your inner strength and grounding. Let yourself feel resilient, like you're standing firm against whatever life throws your way.

"I am capable of living fully, despite the challenges."

Visualize yourself enjoying an activity you love, one that brings you joy and makes you feel alive. Imagine the details, the sounds, the smells, and the feelings that come with doing something that brings fulfillment. When you see yourself in this positive light, you affirm your ability to embrace life on your terms, regardless of the obstacles.

"I am constantly growing, adapting, and learning."

Imagine yourself as a plant or tree that is continuously blossoming. See new leaves and branches sprouting, signifying your progress and adaptation. Even though chronic conditions may bring difficult days, envision yourself steadily growing through each experience, becoming stronger with every challenge.

"I am deserving of love, patience, and kindness—especially from myself."

Picture yourself looking into a mirror and smiling gently at the person looking back. See yourself as someone who deserves all the kindness you give to others. Remind yourself to embrace self-compassion on days when you're not feeling your best, offering yourself the same encouragement you'd give a friend.

Over time, these affirmations and visualizations can transform into a powerful source of comfort, reminding you of your capacity to face challenges with confidence and self-belief.

This practice can help you cultivate an inner support system, one that celebrates your courage and empowers you to handle each day with a positive outlook.

Building Resilience in Daily Routines

Building resilience is an ongoing journey. Resilience isn't just about enduring tough times; it's about adapting and growing through adversity. This growth begins with acknowledging that while challenges are inevitable, our coping strategies can evolve to better manage symptoms.

One effective way to create resilience is by implementing small, consistent practices into daily life. For instance, consider starting each day with a structured morning routine. Establishing such routines offers a sense of predictability and stability, which can be incredibly grounding when facing the unpredictabilities associated with Crohn's disease and ulcerative colitis. Morning rituals might include activities such as gentle stretching, meditation, or simply enjoying a cup of tea in silence; this can set a positive tone for the entire day.

A useful approach might involve writing down your morning plan the night before. This could include setting out clothes, preparing breakfast options, or scheduling time for a brief walk. The objective is to create a sequence of manageable steps that enhance daily life structure.

Engaging in regular physical activities also plays a pivotal role in building resilience. We have already explored how exercising has been shown to boost mood and improve stress management, both of which are crucial for managing health conditions.

However, remember not to embark on this journey alone. Surround yourself with supportive people who understand and empathize with the unique challenges of living with a chronic condition.

As we conclude this chapter on positivity, appreciate the power of gratitude, affirmation, and resilience as allies in facing each day. These practices should remind you of your strength and the light you bring, helping you thrive even in the toughest moments. In the next chapter, we will dive into how you can carry that same spirit into social settings, learning to navigate gatherings, friendships, and daily interactions with ease and confidence.

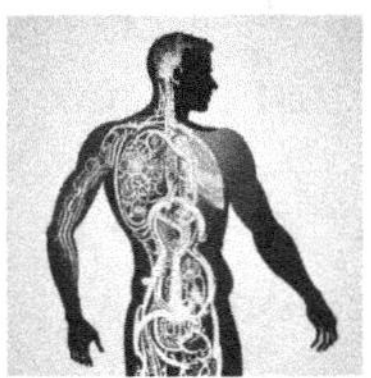

Chapter 7: Social Butterflies— Navigating Life With IBD

B eing in social situations when you have Crohn's disease or ulcerative colitis can sometimes be a little challenging, given that you have to watch your health management, which may oppose your desire to maintain a fulfilling social life. It's important to remember that enjoying time with friends and family can be just as beneficial for mental well-being as managing physical symptoms. Social settings are opportunities for pleasure and empowerment through thoughtful communication.

In this chapter, we will explore practical strategies for thriving socially while addressing the unique needs posed by these chronic conditions. We will look into how clear and honest communication can help manage expectations and create more inclusive environments. Let's get started.

Communicating Needs in Social Settings

When you're living with Crohn's disease or ulcerative colitis, having conversations about your health is a powerful way to create supportive environments and understanding among friends, family, and colleagues. By articulating your needs clearly, you advocate for yourself and open the door for others to understand and support you more effectively.

Imagine this scenario: You've been invited to a friend's dinner party, but you're uncertain about how your body will react on that particular day. You know that your symptoms can sometimes be unpredictable, which might make you hesitant to RSVP. Here's where assertive communication becomes important. Before the event, consider reaching out to the host. Express gratitude for the invitation while also sharing any dietary restrictions or logistical needs you might have. For instance, you could say something like, "I'd love to come to the party, and I appreciate the invite. I want to let you know that my digestive health sometimes complicates things. Is there a quiet place I could step away if needed?"

This approach sets expectations and also empowers your friends and family to provide better support. They're likely to be more accommodating when they truly understand your needs, enhancing their ability to assist and making them more mindful during future gatherings.

Sharing health needs can reduce anxiety and allow social interactions to be more enjoyable. You've likely experienced moments where keeping health concerns to yourself led to unnecessary stress—worrying about potential flare-ups or feeling pressured to explain why you can't partake in certain activities. When you openly communicate, you help put yourself at ease. A simple, honest conversation can alleviate much of the burden, as people often respond with empathy and support.

Normalization doesn't mean broadcasting every detail of your condition to everyone you meet, but rather being open about it in relevant situations. Over time, this can help demystify chronic illnesses for others. When someone asks how you're doing, and it's appropriate to share, you might say, "I'm managing pretty well today, though the recent change in weather has been a bit challenging for my symptoms." Such transparency can spark understanding and make discussions about health issues feel natural and unpressured.

Having some humor in conversations helps break down barriers. While it's essential to gauge the appropriateness based on your audience, a light-hearted comment like, "Well, my intestines decided to throw a surprise party today," can communicate how you're feeling while simultaneously easing tension. This strategy helps maintain a positive atmosphere and shows that while you acknowledge the seriousness of your condition, you're still approaching life with optimism.

If starting these conversations feels challenging, practical strategies could involve preparation and practice. Consider rehearsing what you'd like to say ahead of time, either by jotting down notes or talking it through with a trusted friend or therapist. Having a few key points in mind can boost your confidence when entering these discussions.

Handling Dietary Restrictions Politely

When discussing dietary considerations, it's essential to articulate them in terms that are relatable and empathetic. Instead of diving into medical jargon or complex explanations, frame your needs in ways that others can easily grasp. For instance, you might explain that certain foods are not well tolerated with your gut, similar to how some people avoid spicy foods because they cause discomfort. When you draw parallels to common experiences, you make your needs more relatable, encouraging understanding rather than confusion.

In social settings like dinner parties or gatherings, suggesting dining alternatives can ease potential tension and involve hosts in the conversation about menu planning. Suppose a friend invites you over for a meal. You could mention your dietary preferences and offer to bring a dish or suggest a few options that fit your needs. This approach takes the pressure off the host and encourages open dialogue about how to accommodate everyone's needs without putting anyone on the spot.

In other social settings, It's natural for friends and family to want to share their culinary creations with you, but when these aren't suitable, declining with kindness is key. Phrasing your refusal positively can help—say something like, "That looks amazing, but I'll pass, thank you!" or "I know it's delicious, I'll just stick with what works best for me today." This polite yet firm approach conveys appreciation for the offer while reinforcing your boundaries without offense.

Educating friends on inclusive dining practices for future gatherings can also facilitate smoother social interactions. When friends understand your dietary landscape, they can feel more empowered to contribute to a supportive environment. This education doesn't have to occur right at the event; casual conversations at other times can be beneficial. Sharing articles and recipes or even inviting them to cook together might spark interest and understanding. They'll gain insight into what you can enjoy, which will make hosting you more comfortable for everyone involved.

Feeling empowered to decline invitations without guilt is crucial. You needn't attend every gathering that might put you in a difficult position with regard to your specific diet habits. Politely declining with honesty helps maintain relationships without sacrificing personal well-being. Explaining to the host that while you appreciate the invite, you're prioritizing your health in your decision speaks volumes of self-care. This transparency often leads to solutions where friends may reschedule or modify plans to better suit your needs.

Ultimately, these approaches create a community around you that is aware and accommodating, reducing stress and enabling you to participate fully in social activities. With understanding comes a greater sense of belonging and support from both sides.

For caregivers and family members, being proactive in learning about and accommodating these dietary needs shows empathy and support. Health and wellness professionals can also take these strategies back to their clients, extending the reach of these inclusive practices into broader societal norms.

Navigating Societal Expectations

Society often holds misconceptions, seeing individuals with chronic conditions as constantly unwell or unable to participate fully in social activities. This stereotype can create unnecessary barriers. It's okay to challenge these perceptions by openly discussing chronic diseases in everyday conversations. Doing so raises awareness and also prepares you for potential challenges you might encounter in social settings.

Self-advocacy plays a vital role in reminding yourself that you are not defined solely by your condition. Taking pride in other aspects of oneself and recognizing personal strengths outside your diagnosis is crucial. Engaging in hobbies, cultivating talents, and celebrating achievements helps reinforce this sense of self. These attributes should be highlighted in social scenarios, serving as a reminder to everyone involved that the individual is multifaceted and capable.

Promoting inclusivity within social scenarios involves encouraging friends and acquaintances to recognize the diverse needs of individuals with chronic illnesses. Educating peers about the variability of symptoms and the unpredictability of Crohn's disease and ulcerative colitis creates a more supportive environment. Friends can be allies by asking inclusive questions, offering accommodations when necessary, and respecting each individual's comfort level. This type of consideration allows for more inclusive interventions, expanding social opportunities without causing stress or discomfort.

The power of humor and optimism should not be underestimated in altering stereotypical views and acceptance. Using lightheartedness to deflect negative assumptions demonstrates resilience and reframes chronic conditions as just one part of an enriching life journey. Sharing humorous anecdotes about everyday experiences with chronic conditions can normalize the conversation, showing that laughter and chronic illness can coexist.

In this chapter, we explored how effective communication and understanding can transform the social experiences when living with Crohn's disease and ulcerative colitis. When you articulate your needs, whether it's discussing dietary restrictions or politely declining invitations, you can alleviate social anxiety and foster stronger relationships.

In the next chapter, we will explore different do-it-yourself natural remedies that can help alleviate your symptoms and make living more comfortable.

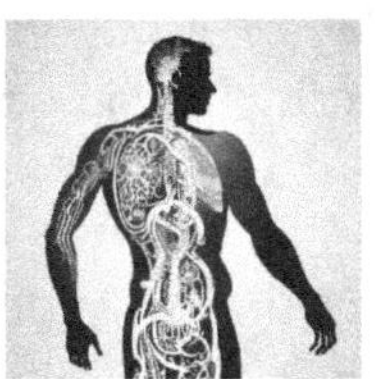

Chapter 8: DIY Remedies and Natural Wonders

Exploring natural remedies offers a refreshing approach to managing the challenges associated with Crohn's disease and ulcerative colitis. With natural complementary methods, you can discover ways to enhance your health and well-being beyond modern medical treatments. Natural remedies provide physical relief and encourage a holistic lifestyle that encompasses both body and mind. This chapter will help you integrate elements from nature into daily routines that can potentially improve your quality of life. I have found these remedies to be beneficial in my journey while living with ulcerative colitis.

Herbal Supplements for Digestive Health

In exploring herbal supplements for digestive health, especially when managing Crohn's disease and ulcerative colitis, we begin with the golden spice, turmeric.

Turmeric: A Golden Elixir for Health

Turmeric is often considered the gold standard of natural anti-inflammatory foods, thanks to its active compound, curcumin. Curcumin is known for its ability to reduce inflammation at the cellular level by blocking inflammatory pathways in the body. This is important when calming the inflammation that irritates the intestinal lining in ulcerative colitis. Turmeric can be easily incorporated into your diet by adding it to curries, soups, teas, or even golden milk—a soothing warm beverage made with plant-based milk and spices. Pairing turmeric with a pinch of black pepper significantly enhances curcumin absorption, making it even more effective.

Ginger

Alongside turmeric, ginger emerges as another potent remedy. Known for its effectiveness in relieving nausea and digestive discomfort, ginger can be soothing during flare-ups of IDB. Ginger's appeal lies in its versatility, as it can be consumed fresh, dried, or as an infusion. It offers a natural way to mitigate symptoms that might otherwise hinder daily activities. During times when digestion is compromised, sipping ginger tea can provide immediate relief, acting as a warm, comforting solution to an unsettled stomach. The anti-nausea properties of ginger are well-documented and have been celebrated in traditional medicine systems across various cultures, reinforcing its place as a staple in managing digestive issues.

Peppermint

Peppermint oil adds an aromatic twist to this collection of herbal remedies. Known for its antispasmodic properties, peppermint oil assists in relieving bloating and cramping, common discomforts associated with Crohn's disease and ulcerative colitis. Beyond physical relief, peppermint oil can aid in providing mental clarity and stress reduction. Stress often exacerbates digestive issues, creating a cycle of discomfort and anxiety. Incorporating peppermint can break this cycle by promoting relaxation while simultaneously soothing the digestive tract. Some find diffusing peppermint oil or incorporating it into massages particularly helpful, merging its calming scent with its therapeutic properties.

Chia Seeds and Flaxseeds

Chia seeds and flaxseeds are small but mighty sources of omega-3 fatty acids. Omega-3s work by balancing inflammatory markers in the body, which can be beneficial for managing the chronic inflammation associated with ulcerative colitis. These seeds are also rich in fiber, promoting healthy digestion and supporting the growth of beneficial gut bacteria. Sprinkle chia seeds into your yogurt, oatmeal, or smoothies, or use flaxseed meal as an egg substitute in baking. For best results, grind flaxseeds before consumption to maximize nutrient absorption.

Herbal Helpers: Anti-Inflammatory Teas

Herbal teas such as chamomile, peppermint, and green tea can complement your anti-inflammatory diet. Chamomile is known for its calming properties, both for the mind and the digestive system, while peppermint can help soothe bloating and gas. Green tea is rich in catechins, powerful antioxidants that may help reduce inflammation and support overall health. Sipping on these teas throughout the day can provide hydration and therapeutic benefits.

Slippery Elm

When consumed, slippery elm coats and calms the gastrointestinal tract, forming a protective layer that can be particularly beneficial during flare-ups. This mucilaginous quality makes it ideal if you have a sensitive stomach, as it protects and aids in the healing process of irritated tissues. Slippery elm powder can easily be mixed with water to create a soothing gruel or tea, presenting a simple yet effective option if you are seeking comfort without complicating your treatment plans.

If you are interested in integrating herbal supplements, starting with these options can offer a gentle introduction to alternative therapies. With each supplement, there's room for personalization based on your preferences and tolerances. A daily dose of turmeric could become part of a morning smoothie, while ginger might be best enjoyed as a midday tea break. Peppermint oil can be an evening ritual, with a few drops added to a diffuser, encouraging relaxation before sleep, and slippery elm might serve as an afternoon pick-me-up in the form of a comforting drink.

When introducing these herbal options to your body, it's essential to integrate them gradually and observe how your system responds. While generally considered safe, some people may experience sensitivity to certain herbs, underscoring the importance of attentive and mindful consumption. It's also beneficial to consult with healthcare professionals before introducing new elements into your routine, especially if you're managing other medications as part of your treatment plan.

Aromatherapy for Relaxation and Symptom Relief

Aromatherapy holds a unique place among natural remedies, offering an opportunity to explore self-care alternatives that promote relaxation and symptom management. Let's explore some aromatherapy options that can help improve your well-being.

Lavender Oil

For centuries, lavender oil has been cherished for its calming properties. This versatile oil can be used in various ways, such as diffusing in a room or applying it topically on the skin. When inhaled, lavender's soothing scent may help reduce the anxiety and tension often associated with chronic health conditions. The act of placing a few drops in a diffuser can transform an environment into a peaceful sanctuary, encouraging tranquility and stress relief. Topical applications, such as massaging diluted lavender oil onto the temples or wrists, can enhance its calming effects, making it an accessible tool for daily stress management.

Chamomile

Another powerful ally in the world of aromatherapy is chamomile, renowned for its ability to aid muscle relaxation and improve sleep quality. Its gentle aroma is often infused into teas and oils, promoting restful sleep and contributing to the body's natural healing processes. When you are experiencing gastrointestinal distress, the relaxing effects of chamomile can be particularly beneficial. You can enjoy its benefits by adding it to nighttime routines, either through a diffuser or a warm bath. This will help you create a bedtime ritual that encourages relaxation and supports digestive comfort.

Eucalyptus Oil

Eucalyptus oil offers invigorating and clarifying benefits, which are especially valuable for respiratory support and reducing anxiety. When diffused, eucalyptus releases a refreshing scent that can help open nasal passages and improve breathing, bringing a sense of relief and ease if you feel overwhelmed or anxious. Embracing eucalyptus oil during moments of stress can provide mental clarity and an energy boost, creating an atmosphere conducive to calmness and comfort, whether at home or in a therapeutic setting.

Frankincense

With its rich history tied to meditation and spiritual practices, frankincense provides emotional relief and positivity. This essential oil enhances focus and tranquility, making it an ideal companion for meditation practices. Incorporating frankincense into meditation can deepen the experience by grounding the mind and creating a state of serenity and introspection. Whether through inhalation or by adding a few drops to a personal altar, frankincense can help facilitate a meditative journey that enriches the spirit and mind.

While essential oils offer diverse benefits, it's important to approach their use with care. Essential oils should always be diluted properly when applied to the skin to prevent irritation, and if you have any specific allergies or sensitivities, you should consult with healthcare professionals before use. Proper guidance ensures these natural remedies are safe and effective, supporting holistic approaches to wellness.

The versatility and accessibility of aromatherapy make it an appealing option for those seeking complementary therapies to manage symptoms associated with Crohn's disease and ulcerative colitis. Aside from addressing physical discomforts, these essential oils offer emotional and mental support, assisting you in navigating life's challenges with increased resilience and optimism.

Incorporating Natural Methods Into Treatment Plans

When you combine herbal supplements with dietary adjustments, aromatherapy, healthcare advice, and a balanced routine, you can maximize your well-being when managing most chronic conditions.

Herbal supplements, when used thoughtfully with dietary adjustments, can yield digestive health benefits. These natural products are rich in bioactive compounds such as flavonoids and essential oils, which are historically recognized for their medicinal properties (Huang et al., 2023). The inclusion of natural fibers and herbs known for their soothing qualities, like slippery elm and psyllium husk, can help in managing digestive discomfort by supporting gut health and reducing inflammation. These supplements help in alleviating symptoms such as bloating and irregular bowel movements and also promote an overall sense of well-being by ensuring proper nutrient absorption. This integration ensures that the body gets the most out of both the herbal supplements and the nutrition provided by a carefully considered diet, enhancing tissue repair and immune function.

Moreover, adopting a balanced routine in line with natural strategies and traditional medical approaches creates comprehensive well-being. Such a routine recognizes the interplay between mind, body, and spirit, creating a lifestyle that supports healing on multiple levels.

Incorporating natural methods doesn't mean disregarding conventional medicine; instead, it highlights the synergy that occurs when both are combined thoughtfully. This blend empowers you with a broader spectrum of tools to manage your condition effectively, emphasizing preventive care and self-awareness.

In this chapter, we have explored natural alternatives such as herbal supplements and aromatherapy, highlighting their potential to enhance your well-being in managing Crohn's disease and ulcerative colitis. Each of these supplements offers unique properties that address discomforts such as inflammation, nausea, and cramping.

In the next chapter, we will explore how you can build a supportive community around you that can offer emotional support to help you navigate your daily symptoms and ease your life.

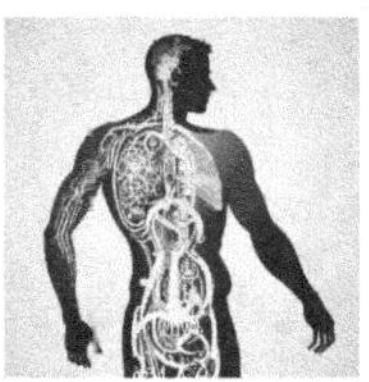

Chapter 9: Building Your Support Squad

Building a support squad is important for managing life's everyday challenges. Having a support group is not merely about assembling a group of people but creating a community that offers understanding and strength in times of need. In this chapter, we will explore how forming connections can transform an often-isolated journey into one enriched with shared wisdom and empathy.

We will look into various strategies to build an invaluable support system and a guide to finding local support groups where you can appreciate face-to-face interactions and create deeper bonds with people going through the same struggles as you. By the end, you'll have a comprehensive understanding of how to create a supportive environment that celebrates collective resilience while addressing your individual needs.

Finding Local Support Groups

Living with Crohn's disease and ulcerative colitis can sometimes feel like an isolating experience, but forming a support squad through local groups can transform this journey into one filled with empathy and understanding. Support groups offer immense emotional benefits, providing safe spaces where sharing personal stories is welcome and encouraged. You may find relief in knowing that others genuinely understand your challenges without the need for extensive explanations. This mutual understanding reduces feelings of isolation and fosters connections built on shared experiences.

Being part of a group also means having access to diverse perspectives and coping strategies, which is empowering. For instance, hearing about how someone else manages flare-ups or dietary restrictions might offer a new perspective you hadn't considered.

Finding these groups might seem challenging at first, but there are several clear paths to discovery. One effective way is through hospitals and health organizations, which often host or partner with support groups to provide comprehensive care. Additionally, directories from foundations such as the Crohn's & Colitis Foundation offer listings of available groups, making it easier to find one close to home. These resources are invaluable if you are willing to connect with others facing similar health journeys.

When exploring the world of support groups, it helps to know what to expect during meetings. Typically, these gatherings are informal and friendly, designed to put everyone at ease. Meeting formats can vary—some may focus on open discussions while others offer structured activities or guest speakers. The dynamic nature of these settings allows attendees to exchange resources, whether it's tips on managing symptoms or information about the latest treatments. Empowerment flourishes when you view yourself as an engaged contributor rather than a passive receiver of guidance.

Preparing discussion topics ahead of time can help ensure you're contributing meaningfully. Sharing your own stories and challenges can benefit you by creating an outlet and also aids fellow members who might gain strength from your courage. Remember, it's not just about receiving support but also offering it, thus enhancing the communal bond within the group.

Furthermore, building relationships beyond meetings can enhance your support network. Consider following up with new friends to nurture these connections outside of designated group times. This may be via text, phone calls, or casual meetups. Maintaining contact reinforces the sense of community and shared journey. Having people who truly understand your day-to-day struggles and triumphs can provide comfort and encouragement long after the meeting ends.

Another strategy involves setting personal goals for each session. Before attending, think about what you hope to achieve—whether it's gaining new knowledge, finding solutions to specific problems, or simply connecting with someone who gets it. This purposeful approach ensures that each meeting is both relevant and rewarding to your unique needs.

To further your engagement, consider taking on a leadership role within the group over time. Facilitating discussions or organizing events could deepen your involvement and create bigger impacts. There's something satisfying about contributing to the well-being of others while enriching your own life.

Utilizing Online Communities Wisely

Online communities are virtual spaces where individuals who share similar experiences connect and provide access to information and resources that might otherwise be hard to come by. However, engaging with these communities requires thoughtful consideration to maximize your benefits while avoiding potential pitfalls.

Identifying Reputable Online Platforms

When searching for online support groups, selecting reputable platforms is crucial. Look for forums or social media groups that have established moderation protocols to ensure content is accurate and interactions are respectful. Platforms associated with credible health organizations, such as the Crohn's & Colitis Foundation, often adhere to guidelines that promote constructive discussion and discourage misinformation. These spaces typically have knowledgeable moderators or health professionals available to field questions, adding an extra layer of trustworthiness. When you choose well-monitored communities, you're more likely to find reliable information and positive interactions that contribute to your healing process.

Another aspect to consider when identifying platforms is community engagement. Thriving online communities often encourage active participation through regular updates, webinars, and Q&A sessions that enrich the member experience. Many feature testimonies from healthcare professionals or patients who are successfully managing their symptoms, providing both inspiration and practical advice. Take the time to explore different groups to find one that resonates with you, where members share a genuine interest in learning and supporting each other.

Establishing Boundaries

While connecting with others online can be rewarding, it is important to establish boundaries to maintain a healthy balance between digital interaction and personal life. Set limits on how much time you spend within these communities; this will help prevent burnout and stress. It's easy to lose track of time on social media, which may inadvertently add to the anxiety rather than alleviate your symptoms. Decide on specific times during the day or week to engage with your chosen group, ensuring that your involvement remains sustainable.

Another important boundary is being selective about the type of information you absorb. Focus on content that offers constructive advice, encouragement, and factual insights into managing Crohn's and colitis. Avoid posts that stir negativity or alarm, as these can exacerbate feelings of helplessness or fear. Engage in discussions that uplift and educate, contributing positively to your mental well-being. Remember, quality over quantity is key when curating your online support experience.

Sharing Experiences Thoughtfully

When it comes to sharing your journey, a thoughtful approach is vital. It's important to consider the mental health implications of publicizing your personal experiences. Reflect on what you're comfortable sharing; keep in mind that the internet has a wide reach. Prioritize maintaining personal privacy by being cautious about disclosing detailed medical information or identifying characteristics unless you're confident in the security of the platform and the intentions of its users.

Sharing coping strategies, treatment successes, or lifestyle adaptations can offer valuable insights to others facing similar challenges. This creates a sense of solidarity and also reinforces your journey by opening avenues for new ideas and solutions.

Connecting Beyond Online Platforms

While the digital world provides a convenient way to meet others with Crohn's and colitis, transforming these connections into real-life support networks can enhance the overall experience. Organizing meetups or local gatherings enables you to build deeper relationships, offering the emotional reassurance that physical presence can bring. Whether it's meeting for coffee or attending health-related workshops together, these interactions emphasize shared understanding and camaraderie.

Social media can be instrumental in facilitating local connections. Utilize features like location tagging or event pages to identify peers in your geographic area and arrange informal get-togethers. Engaging in activities outside the digital space broadens your network and introduces opportunities to exchange tangible resources, such as recommendations for doctors, diet plans, or wellness programs.

Building a Diverse Support Network

Integrating local support groups and online communities can significantly enhance your support system when dealing with Crohn's Disease and Ulcerative Colitis.

Local support groups provide face-to-face interaction and a sense of camaraderie that is often hard to replicate online. These interactions help build trust and understanding among group members through shared experiences and emotional support. Such gatherings allow you to receive care and empathy and also offer an opportunity to help others by sharing your journey, thereby creating a fulfilling loop of support.

On the flip side, online communities bring together individuals from diverse backgrounds and geographic locations, offering a broader perspective on managing life with these conditions. Engaging in forums, social media groups, and virtual meetups expands your reach beyond physical limitations, giving you access to varied insights and experiences. Online spaces are often available 24/7, providing immediate support during times of need or crisis and enabling continuous learning about new coping mechanisms or medical advancements.

The goal is to seamlessly blend these environments into a cohesive support system that evolves alongside you. Integrate regular participation in both settings, ensuring you remain informed about the latest strategies and treatments. In local groups, you might find solace in discussing personal concerns, whereas online platforms might introduce you to alternative therapies or emerging research. This combination nurtures adaptability and ensures you're always equipped with the knowledge to tackle challenges head-on.

Using digital tools effectively can bridge any existing gaps between these two worlds. Video calls, instant messaging apps, and social media platforms can maintain connections with local friends even outside scheduled meetings. By using these tools creatively, meaningful discussions started in one setting can continue in another, promoting continuity and collaboration. For instance, a WhatsApp group formed after an in-person meeting can facilitate ongoing conversations, allowing members to share articles and personal victories, or seek advice between sessions.

Witnessing how others cope can inspire strength and ingenuity, helping you navigate your journey with increased confidence and optimism.

As your network grows, so does the potential to raise awareness, campaign for better healthcare policies, or drive research funding. This collective voice can have a lasting impact, influencing public perception and enhancing the lives of everyone touched by Crohn's and colitis.

As we close this chapter, we've explored the transformative role that building a community can play in navigating life with Crohn's disease and ulcerative colitis. Through finding local support groups, you can gain emotional relief and also invaluable insights and strategies from those who truly understand your journey. Remember to lean on your support team—they're invaluable. Whether it's a conversation in a Facebook group or reaching out to your hospital team, these connections can provide the encouragement and guidance that help you keep moving forward.

In the next chapter, we will look into how you can celebrate your gut journey as you reflect on your progress and be proud of the milestones you are setting up for the future.

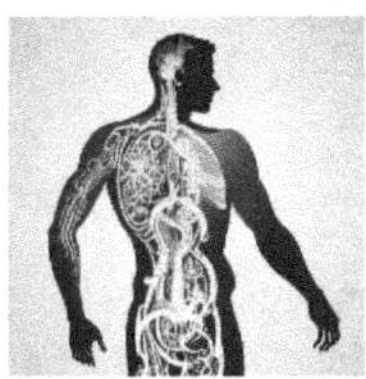

Chapter 10:
Celebrating Your Gut Journey

Acknowledging the journey of gut health is more than tracking symptoms; it's about celebrating progress and setting sights on future successes. This chapter invites you to recognize the importance of reflecting on your path and understanding that every small victory contributes to a broader picture of well-being. We will look at various ways to celebrate your progress and how you may set inspiring future goals.

Journaling Milestones of Success

In the journey to better gut health, we have already talked about how it is important to track your progress. This helps you acknowledge your achievements over time and also lays the groundwork for future success. Having a daily log is one of the most effective ways to track your progress.

At its core, a daily log serves as a resource for identifying patterns and triggers related to Crohn's disease and ulcerative colitis. By documenting daily symptoms, dietary intake, and physical activities, you can begin to discern what works for you and what doesn't. For instance, if you note persistent discomfort after consuming certain foods, these recordings become instrumental in pinpointing dietary triggers. Over time, this methodical documentation helps create a deeper understanding of your body and how it reacts to different scenarios. Moreover, maintaining a regular log opens up a chance for self-discovery. It invites you to engage with your health on a more profound level.

Furthermore, sharing personal logs with healthcare providers significantly enhances management and treatment plans. Doctors can offer more targeted advice when they have comprehensive data about your daily experiences. For example, if a gastroenterologist reviews a month's worth of logs, they might notice correlations between stress levels and symptom severity, leading to more tailored treatment strategies. This collaborative approach empowers you and healthcare providers to work together effectively.

To create an effective daily log, use whichever medium feels most comfortable—this can be a dedicated app, notebook, or computer document. Begin each day by jotting down significant details: meals consumed, any notable symptoms, activities engaged in, and overall mood. As the days turn into weeks and weeks into months, patterns will inevitably emerge, painting a clearer picture of your health journey.

Planning Rewarding Activities for Achievements

Celebrating progress on your gut health journey is about infusing joy and gratitude into every step forward. When living with conditions like Crohn's disease or ulcerative colitis, it's essential to focus on the challenges and also on small victories that mark your growth. Introducing a reward system aligned with achievements is a powerful motivator. Simple pleasures, such as treating yourself to your favorite meal when dietary limitations allow or enjoying a new book, serve as badges of honor for your efforts. The key is to make these rewards personal and meaningful, ensuring they resonate with your passions and interests. Let's look into fun ways to celebrate your milestones.

Self-Care

Creating self-care days dedicated entirely to relaxation can reinforce this rewarding experience. Self-care days are more than just indulgences; they're a vital part of maintaining mental health. Taking time to relax helps you recharge, offering a break from the rigorous routines of your daily life. Self-care can include activities such as soaking in a warm bath, practicing gentle yoga, or meditating. This allows you to listen to your body's needs and respond with kindness. Regularly scheduling these days reminds you to prioritize well-being, preventing burnout, and keeping stress at bay.

Social Celebration

Milestones on your health journey become more significant when shared with loved ones. This may be hosting a small gathering with friends after a successful check-up or sharing a special dinner with family to celebrate reduced symptoms; these moments solidify bonds and foster relationships. Such gatherings create a sense of community, transforming individual triumphs into collective cheer.

Social celebrations also open up a dialogue about your journey, which can cultivate empathy and understanding among those around you. When you include others in your celebrations, you're recognizing your achievements and also educating them about the nuances of living with your condition. This creates a supportive network that can offer encouragement and companionship during more challenging times.

Capture the Moment With Photos

Each milestone you reach is part of your larger story, so why not document it? Consider creating a personal photo journal or even a digital album where you record each accomplishment. You can take photos, write down your thoughts, or add little mementos—anything that captures the moment. Revisiting these memories can give you motivation on tough days, reminding you of how far you've come.

Give Back to Others

One of the most meaningful ways to celebrate can be to share your progress with others. If you're part of an online or in-person support group, share your success story and insights. Celebrate by volunteering, starting a small fundraiser, or simply offering encouragement to someone else on a similar journey. By giving back, you reinforce the strength within you and help build a supportive community around your shared experiences.

Nonetheless, it's vital to balance these joyful experiences with realism. Celebrations should never feel like obligations or add pressure to an already demanding routine. Instead, they should serve as positive affirmations of progress, no matter how gradual.

Creating Vision Boards

Embarking on a journey to improve gut health while managing Crohn's disease and ulcerative colitis is no small feat. It's a path that requires motivation, resilience, and perseverance. A vision board is a powerful tool that can help you maintain these qualities.

Vision boards are more than just collages; they are daily reminders of our aspirations and achievements. They serve as a constant visual stimulus that keeps our goals at the forefront of our minds. It helps maintain an optimistic outlook even when faced with the inevitable challenges associated with your condition. A well-constructed vision board can remind you of the progress you've made and the potential that still lies ahead, helping to create a sense of accomplishment and positivity.

The beauty of creating a vision board lies in its process as much as its outcome. It's an opportunity to engage creatively and expressively, giving life to dreams and hopes. Involving family and friends in this process can add support and encouragement. Assembling a vision board with loved ones creates a shared experience and allows them to contribute their understanding and empathy. This inclusion is particularly beneficial during tough times, where collective encouragement becomes a beacon of hope. Friends and family members participating in this creative endeavor can offer insights or remind us of past accomplishments, further boosting morale.

Encouragement from vision boards communicates a narrative of triumph over adversity—even when setbacks occur. Each image or word placed on a board represents a step forward, no matter how small. Seeing these positive affirmations regularly can help instill hope, reinforcing the idea that challenges do not define the journey but rather punctuate it. This realization is empowering. It reassures you that despite the hurdles, progress is tangible and achievable.

Inspiring Future Goals

The following are some inspiring future goals you may use for your vision board. If you have no clue how to begin, these ideas are crafted to cultivate a sense of purpose and inspiration within you as you face the future.

Visualize Your Ideal Future

You can start by picturing your life in an ideal world—what does it look like? How are you spending your time, and who's with you along the way? You may envision a lifestyle where you're confidently managing IBD, enjoying fulfilling relationships, pursuing meaningful work, or exploring hobbies that bring you joy. Let this vision guide your goals; remember, it's not about perfection but creating a life that feels satisfying and intentional.

Break Down Goals Into Manageable Steps

Large goals can feel daunting, but breaking them down into smaller, achievable steps can make them feel doable. For instance, if you aim to build physical strength, start with a gentle fitness routine that gradually increases in intensity. If your goal is to improve nutrition, begin by incorporating one new healthy habit at a time—like trying one gut-friendly recipe each week or learning more about the foods that work best for you.

Each small step will build momentum, and as you progress, you'll see how these small actions add up to meaningful change.

Set Goals Aligned With Your Well-Being

When living with IBD, wellness-centered goals often have the most lasting impact. These might include prioritizing stress management, developing a reliable sleep routine, or finding exercise options that work with your body's needs. Goals focused on overall well-being are incredibly empowering; they put you in control of your health in ways that support and enhance your quality of life.

Cultivate Long-Term Personal Passions

Part of creating inspiring future goals includes setting intentions that go beyond managing health. When you focus on personal interests and passions, you remind yourself that life is full of opportunities for growth and enjoyment. You may want to start a creative hobby, learn a new skill, or take steps toward a career or volunteer role that feels meaningful to you.

Whatever your passions, these goals encourage a mindset shift: instead of focusing solely on managing symptoms, you're working toward a fulfilling life that's meaningful to you.

Concluding Thoughts

Acknowledging progress and setting future goals are essential steps in maintaining motivation and resilience on your gut health journey.

By celebrating small victories, privately and with loved ones, you will strengthen bonds and fortify a sense of accomplishment. Tools like vision boards serve as constant reminders of goals, bolstering optimism even during setbacks. These visual aids, together with rewarding activities, inspire perseverance and create a narrative of triumph over adversity. Through this chapter, it's evident that clarity, consistency, and celebration are pillars of resilience. They transform the path toward improved health into one marked by hope, adaptability, and shared successes.

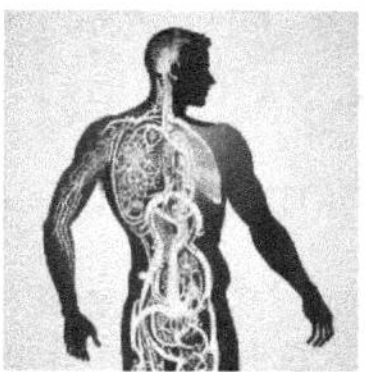

Conclusion

As we conclude this exploration into living with Crohn's disease and ulcerative colitis, let's reflect on the journey we've embarked upon together. This book has guided you through understanding your condition from multiple perspectives—shedding light on microbiomes, nutrition, stress, exercise, medication, positivity, social interaction, natural remedies, support systems, and celebrating achievements. We uncovered how crucial it is to recognize that your microbiome is more than just a collection of tiny organisms; it's an ally in managing these conditions. Nourishing your body with the right foods can serve as fuel for your daily battles, empowering you to overcome the toughest challenges with resilience and strength.

We've seen the importance of choosing foods that provide sustenance and also partner with your gut in promoting health and reducing flare-ups. From there, stress management emerged as another pivotal point. We explored techniques for calming your mind and finding balance amidst the chaos these diseases can sometimes bring.

We also explored how exercises play a significant role in maintaining well-being. Whether it's yoga, swimming, or a gentle stroll in the park, moving your body is a testament to your commitment to staying above these conditions. Alongside physical activity, various medications help manage symptoms and prevent complications. Understanding your medication plan, including potential side effects, equips you with the knowledge to make informed decisions regarding your treatment.

We also delved into the transformative power of positivity. Challenges are inevitable, yet viewing them through a lens of optimism can alter your experience entirely. Laughter, humor, and joy have their place in healing—easing discomforts and bringing light to even the darkest days. We also explored how you can handle social situations, especially setups that can compromise your diet plan.

We covered natural remedies as effective supplements to conventional treatments. Herbal teas, probiotics, and acupuncture might not be the perfect fit for everyone, but they provide additional options worth considering under professional guidance. Furthermore, we explored how surrounding yourself with a supportive network fosters connectedness that uplifts your spirit. Whether friends, family, or fellow warriors in support groups, building relationships with people who understand your journey offers comfort and camaraderie. We went on to look into why it is important to celebrate your achievements, no matter how small. Acknowledging progress strengthens your resolve and keeps your motivation high.

Your experiences are individual, laced with lessons specific to your life. No two paths are identical, but each is valuable. Celebrate your individuality and resilience in confronting Crohn's and colitis. Allow yourself grace amid setbacks, and champion your victories, however modest they seem.

Maintaining a positive outlook doesn't mean ignoring difficulties or pretending everything is perfect. Instead, cultivate a hopeful mindset while staying vigilant about your health. Be proactive—set realistic goals, track progress, and address concerns promptly. Consider your health journey akin to tending a garden. With attentive care like watering, weeding, and nurturing, you'll cultivate a thriving harvest of well-being. Invest daily in positivity, spread seeds of optimism, and take time to appreciate the blossoms along the way.

Remember, there's no single formula for living with Crohn's and colitis. It's a balancing act, constantly adjusting based on new information, experiences, and personal growth. Continue exploring, learning, and adapting.

As we close, remember that you're capable, resilient, and never alone in your pursuit of health and happiness. Here's to your continued journey, rich in discovery, support, and fulfillment. I hope this journey through Crohn's and colitis has been both informative and uplifting, showing you that there's hope and even a bit of humor along the way! Remember, support is always available if you need it—you're never alone. With ongoing medical advancements, this journey continues to evolve, bringing more possibilities for patients to find their paths to well-being and resilience.

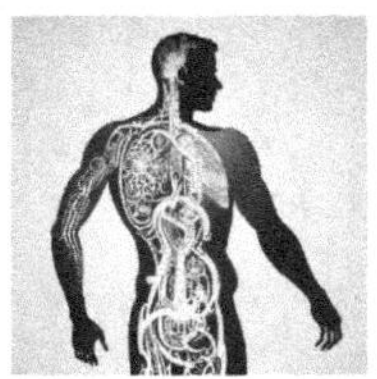

References

Akimbekov, N. S., & Razzaque, M. S. (2021). Laughter therapy: A humor-induced hormonal intervention to reduce stress and anxiety. *Current Research in Physiology, 4*(4), 135–138. https://doi.org/10.1016/j.crphys.2021.04.002

Aslam, N., Lo, S. W., Sikafi, R., Barnes, T., Segal, J., Smith, P. J., & Limdi, J. K. (2022). A review of the therapeutic management of ulcerative colitis. *Therapeutic Advances in Gastroenterology, 15*, 175628482211381. https://doi.org/10.1177/17562848221138160

Bandopadhyay, P., & Ganguly, D. (2022). Gut dysbiosis and metabolic diseases. *Progress in Molecular Biology and Translational Science, 191*(1), 153–174. https://doi.org/10.1016/bs.pmbts.2022.06.031

Bilski, J., Brzozowski, B., Mazur-Bialy, A., Sliwowski, Z., & Brzozowski, T. (2014). The role of physical exercise in inflammatory bowel disease. *BioMed Research International, 2014*, 429031. https://doi.org/10.1155/2014/429031

Cloyd, J. (2023, October 16). *Top 10 herbs for intestinal inflammation.* Rupa Health. https://www.rupahealth.com/post/top-10-herbs-for-intestinal-inflammation

De Sousa, J. F. M., Paghdar, S., Khan, T. M., Patel, N. P., Chandrasekaran, S., & Tsouklidis, N. (2022). Stress and inflammatory bowel disease: Clear mind, happy colon. *Cureus.* https://doi.org/10.7759/cureus.25006

Fekete, E. M., & Deichert, N. T. (2022). A brief gratitude writing intervention decreased stress and negative affect during the COVID-19 pandemic. *Journal of Happiness Studies, 23*(6). https://doi.org/10.1007/s10902-022-00505-6

Forbes, L., & Johnson, S. K. (2022). Online Mindfulness Intervention for Inflammatory Bowel Disease: Adherence and Efficacy. *Frontiers in Psychology, 12.* https://doi.org/10.3389/fpsyg.2021.709899

Godala, M., Gaszyńska, E., Durko, Ł., & Małecka-Wojciesko, E. (2023). Dietary Behaviors and Beliefs in Patients with Inflammatory Bowel Disease. *Journal of Clinical Medicine, 12*(10), 3455. https://doi.org/10.3390/jcm12103455

Hoogkamer, A. B., Brooks, A. J., Rowse, G., & Lobo, A. J. (2020). Predicting the development of psychological morbidity in inflammatory bowel disease: A systematic review. *Frontline Gastroenterology*, flgastro-2019-101353. https://doi.org/10.1136/flgastro-2019-101353

Ju, L., Ke, F., & Yadav, P. (2012). Herbal medicine in the treatment of ulcerative colitis. *Saudi Journal of Gastroenterology, 18*(1), 3. https://doi.org/10.4103/1319-3767.91726

Karimi, N., Moore, A. R., Lukin, A., Kanazaki, R., Williams, A.-J., & Connor, S. (2020). Clinical communication in inflammatory bowel disease: A systematic literature review protocol. *BMJ Open, 10*(11), e039503. https://doi.org/10.1136/bmjopen-2020-039503

Nelson, A. (2024, May 29). *Probiotics, prebiotics, and synbiotics for UC*. WebMD. https://www.webmd.com/ibd-crohns-disease/ulcerative-colitis/ulcerative-colitis-probiotics-prebiotics

Osso, M., & Riehl, M. (2024, August 7). *Stress and IBD: Breaking the vicious cycle*. Crohn's & Colitis Foundation. https://www.crohnscolitisfoundation.org/blog/stress-and-ibd-breaking-the-vicious-cycle

Pitocchelli-Schwartzman, S. (2024, May 15). *Exercise & IBD: A guide for Crohn's & ulcerative colitis | evinature*. Evinature. https://evinature.com/blog/gut-health/ibd-exercise/

Robertson, R. (2017, June 27). *Why the gut microbiome is crucial for your health*. Healthline. https://www.healthline.com/nutrition/gut-microbiome-and-health

Ruwa, R. (2024, June 27). *What is an IBD journal and how can it help?* Healthline; Healthline Media. https://www.healthline.com/health/ibd/ibd-journal

Seladi-Schulman, J. (2021, June 2). *Can essential oils help with Crohn's disease?* Healthline; Healthline Media. https://www.healthline.com/health/crohns-disease/crohns-disease-essential-oils

Sirois, F. M., & Wood, A. M. (2017). Gratitude uniquely predicts lower depression in chronic illness populations: A longitudinal study of inflammatory bowel disease and arthritis. *Health Psychology, 36*(2), 122–132. https://doi.org/10.1037/hea0000436

Smith, R. P., Easson, C., Lyle, S. M., Kapoor, R., Donnelly, C. P., Davidson, E. J., Parikh, E., Lopez, J. V., & Tartar, J. L. (2019). Gut microbiome diversity is associated with sleep physiology in humans. *PLoS ONE, 14*(10). https://doi.org/10.1371/journal.pone.0222394

Szeto, J., Noejovich, C. V., Verma, R., Miranda, P., M Pinto-Sanchez, Verdu, E., & Armstrong, D. (2024). A265 barriers to dietary modification in inflammatory bowel disease (IBD): a mixed-methods assessment of patient perceptions. *Journal of the Canadian Association of Gastroenterology*, *7*(Supplement_1), 213–214. https://doi.org/10.1093/jcag/gwad061.265

Terry, N., & Margolis, K. G. (2017). Serotonergic mechanisms regulating the GI tract: Experimental evidence and therapeutic relevance. *Handbook of Experimental Pharmacology*, *239*, 319–342. https://doi.org/10.1007/164_2016_103

Trindade, I. A., & Sirois, F. M. (2021). The prospective effects of self-compassion on depressive symptoms, anxiety, and stress: A study in inflammatory bowel disease. *Journal of Psychosomatic Research*, 110429. https://doi.org/10.1016/j.jpsychores.2021.110429

Vakadaris, G., Stefanis, C., Giorgi, E., Brouvalis, M., Voidarou, C. (Chrysa), Kourkoutas, Y., Tsigalou, C., & Bezirtzoglou, E. (2023). The role of probiotics in inducing and maintaining remission in Crohn's disease and ulcerative colitis: A systematic review of the literature. *Biomedicines*, *11*(2), 494. https://doi.org/10.3390/biomedicines11020494

Valdes, A. M., Walter, J., Segal, E., & Spector, T. D. (2018). Role of the gut microbiota in nutrition and health. *BMJ*, *361*(361), k2179. https://doi.org/10.1136/bmj.k2179

Watson, S. (2024, May 3). *Manage your stress to ease ulcerative colitis.* WebMD. https://www.webmd.com/ibd-crohns-disease/ulcerative-colitis/uc-relaxation

Wei, L., Singh, R., Ro, S., & Ghoshal, U. C. (2021). Gut microbiota dysbiosis in functional gastrointestinal disorders: Underpinning the symptoms and pathophysiology. *JGH Open*, *5*(9). https://doi.org/10.1002/jgh3.12528

Wu, H.-J., & Wu, E. (2012). The role of gut microbiota in immune homeostasis and autoimmunity. *Gut Microbes*, *3*(1), 4–14. https://doi.org/10.4161/gmic.19320

Zahavi, M. (2015, March 16). *Maintaining an attitude of gratitude with chronic illness: Positive thinking in Crohn's patients*. ResearchGate. https://doi.org/10.13140/RG.2.2.36113.79204